Delivering Person-Centred Care in Nursing

Bob Price

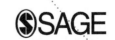

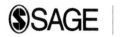

Learning Matters
An imprint of SAGE Publications Ltd
1 Oliver's Yard
55 City Road
London EC1Y 1SP

SAGE Publications Inc.
2455 Teller Road
Thousand Oaks, California 91320

SAGE Publications India Pvt Ltd
B 1/I 1 Mohan Cooperative Industrial Area
Mathura Road
New Delhi 110 044

SAGE Publications Asia-Pacific Pte Ltd
3 Church Street
#10-04 Samsung Hub
Singapore 049483

Editor: Donna Goddard
Development editor: Sarah Turpie
Senior project editor: Chris Marke
Project management: Swales & Willis Ltd, Exeter, Devon
Marketing manager: George Kimble
Cover design: Wendy Scott
Typeset by: C&M Digitals (P) Ltd, Chennai, India
Printed in the UK

Library of Congress Control Number: 2018965492

British Library Cataloguing in Publication Data

A catalogue record for this book is available from the British Library

ISBN 978-1-5264-6333-3
ISBN 978-1-5264-6334-0 (pbk)

At SAGE we take sustainability seriously. Most of our products are printed in the UK using responsibly sourced papers and boards. When we print overseas we ensure sustainable papers are used as measured by the PREPS grading system. We undertake an annual audit to monitor our sustainability.

Delivering Person-Centred Care in Nursing

Sara Miller McCune founded SAGE Publishing in 1965 to support the dissemination of usable knowledge and educate a global community. SAGE publishes more than 1000 journals and over 800 new books each year, spanning a wide range of subject areas. Our growing selection of library products includes archives, data, case studies and video. SAGE remains majority owned by our founder and after her lifetime will become owned by a charitable trust that secures the company's continued independence.

Los Angeles | London | New Delhi | Singapore | Washington DC | Melbourne

Contents

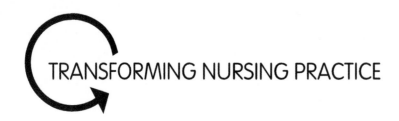

TRANSFORMING NURSING PRACTICE

Transforming Nursing Practice is a series tailor made for pre-registration students nurses.
Each book in the series is:

 Affordable

 Full of active
learning features

 Mapped to the NMC Standards of
proficiency for registered nurses

 Focused on applying
theory to practice

Each book addresses a core topic and they have been carefully developed
to be simple to use, quick to read and written in clear language.

An invaluable series of books that explicitly relates to the NMC standards. Each book covers a different topic that students need to explore in order to develop into a qualified nurse... I would recommend this series to all Pre-Registered nursing students whatever their field or year of study.

LINDA ROBSON,
Senior Lecturer at Edge Hill University

Many titles in the series are on our recommended reading list and for good reason - the content is up to date and easy to read. These are the books that actually get used beyond training and into your nursing career.

EMMA LYDON,
Adult Student Nursing

ABOUT THE SERIES EDITORS

DR MOOI STANDING is an Independent Nursing Consultant (UK and International) and is responsible for the core knowledge, adult nursing and personal and professional learning skills titles. She is an experienced NMC Quality Assurance Reviewer of educational programmes and a Professional Regulator Panellist on the NMC Practice Committee. Mooi is also Board member of Special Olympics Malaysia, enabling people with intellectual disabilities to participate in sports and athletics nationally and internationally.

DR SANDRA WALKER is a Clinical Academic in Mental Health working between Southern Health Trust and the University of Southampton and responsible for the mental health nursing titles. She is a Qualified Mental Health Nurse with a wide range of clinical experience spanning more than 25 years.

BESTSELLING TEXTBOOKS

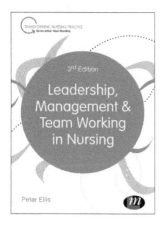

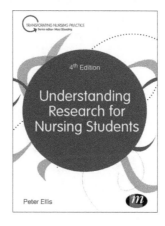

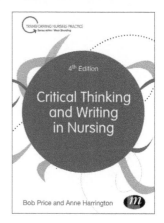

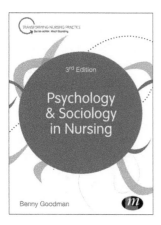

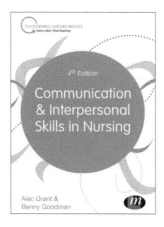

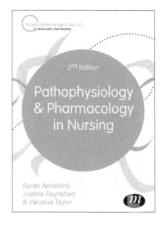

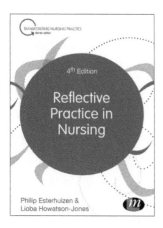

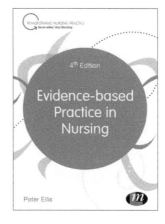

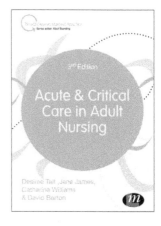

You can find a full list of textbooks in the
Transforming Nursing Practice series at
https://uk.sagepub.com

Foreword

Delivering Person-Centred Care in Nursing is a most welcome addition to the Transforming Nursing Practice series because it puts into words the excellent care nurses aspire to provide but often find difficult to explain. In developing and maintaining our professional identities as nurses, it is important that we can articulate, celebrate and emulate good practice in caring for patients and other service users. If we are unable to do so, there is a danger that the knowledge or skills associated with high standards of person-centred nursing care remain hidden, not fully understood, or not valued as highly as other clinical treatments.

The book tackles the problem by presenting an innovative, structured, pragmatic approach to person-centred nursing care which is easy to follow, relate to, and apply to practice. The stages range from anticipating concerns, to learning lessons which can be easily applied alongside other problem solving approaches from assessment to evaluation. The pragmatic approach offers guidance in how to tune in to the patient's world and collaborate with them to decide what is going on, what needs to happen, and who does what in achieving this. The second stage 'Hearing the patient narrative to understand perceptions' sums up the central importance of understanding the patient's experience. Six chapters are devoted to exploring in-depth real life case studies, demonstrating both the sensitive and challenging nature of delivering pragmatic person-centred nursing care within the different nursing pathways. The book concludes by relating person-centred nursing to future health policy challenges, in addressing the nation's increasing demands for healthcare with limited resources. It is argued that patients' healthcare experience should be researched more as it can provide a wealth of information in how to deliver person-centred care. The need to attend to patients' narratives, to reveal and respond to their personal stories is highlighted in this respect, and linked to greater patient satisfaction with healthcare, and greater job satisfaction for nurses.

This book will help readers to achieve NMC standards of proficiency for registered nurses, for example, *Platform 1: Being an accountable professional – providing nursing care that is person-centred, safe and compassionate* (NMC, 2018a, p7). Likewise, it helps readers to meet NMC Code requirements, for example, *Prioritise people – 2: Listen to people and respond to their preferences and concerns* (NMC, 2018b, p6). It recognises that people can vary from passive recipients to proactive self carers, and a range of nursing roles (problem analyst, counsellor, educator, confidant, motivator) are described in matching what patients need, what they want, and what nurses can offer within an appropriate working partnership. In doing so, it cleverly links good person-centred care with sound evidence-based practice by use of qualitative case studies and narrative research. I highly commend this insightful book to both nursing students and registered nurses negotiating NMC revalidation requirements.

Dr Mooi Standing, Series Editor

About the author

Bob Price is a healthcare education and training consultant. He started his clinical work as a nurse in trauma and then cancer care, developing new ways to address the altered body image needs of patients. Subsequently he led education programmes at the Royal Marsden Hospital (London), the RCN and the Open University. He has been a visiting lecturer to institutes within the UK, Europe and North America. Bob is also a co-author of the SAGE text, *Critical Thinking and Writing in Nursing*.

Acknowledgements

No textbook comes from an author alone. There are editors and critical readers who offer wise counsel, so my sincere thanks to Donna Goddard, Sarah Turpie and Mooi Standing and to the many other colleagues with whom I tried out draft ideas en route. Thank you as well to my wife Adrienne who was allegedly driven to the golf club by my writing.

Introduction

Who is this book for?

This textbook is written for students learning how to nurse. But it will be of value too to registered nurses who are re-evaluating their work. The difference between ideal care and that deliverable today is widely felt. The book refers to a range of care environments, including those serving people with physical and mental health problems, those dealing with learning disability challenges, the very young and the old as well. While divisions of care are used for course teaching, person-centred care transcends all areas of practice. The principles of attending to patient perceptions and narratives (felt situation and need), as well as to clinical or risk needs, remains valuable everywhere. The book is firmly about 'how to' proceed.

Why *Delivering Person-Centred Care*?

One of the greatest challenges within nursing is learning how to deliver care to patients in such a way that it seems both personal and realistic given service constraints. Nursing care is both a process (something negotiated with the patient) and a product (something that the consumer judges the service by) (Kim, 2015). While much of nursing philosophy emphasises that which is highly personal and contracted with the practitioner, much else within healthcare centres on product standards, protocols and policies (Olkiewicz and Bober, 2015). The needs of a nurse (to act in profession-expressive ways) are sometimes in competition with the requirements of a service. Perceptions of need, priority and service sometimes conflict.

In some areas of healthcare work there may be considerable scope to individualise care in ways that are clearly person-centred. There is time for the care relationship to develop (Bartol, 2014). Nurses learn how the patient reasons, what they value or desire. In other care areas, however, such as acute care within hospitals, it may be harder to deliver person-centred care. In these areas there is a greater emphasis on standard care pathways and risk management and less scope to explore different care possibilities (Wood and Garner, 2012). Irrespective of which care environment the nurse practises within, however, the NMC Code of Conduct (*The Code*) requires that patients are treated with respect (Nursing and Midwifery Council (NMC), 2015). The nurse must respect patients as individuals. Person-centred care is much more than politeness.

Because nurses must attend both to the patient as an individual and also work well within a healthcare system, the question arises as to how best might we ensure that care is person-centred? The effective choices open to patients may be quite limited. While patients retain the power of consent, they might not have a range of treatment or support options to choose from. The NHS limits possibilities on the basis of that which can be afforded by the public purse (Oliver, 2017). However, while choices may be limited, the manner in which care is received still provides person-centred care opportunities. It is still possible to relate considerately to patients, even within a system that necessarily standardises much of its provision. That is the subject of this book. We explore ways of relating to patients, communicating with them and supporting them that help them to feel that their care is dignified. We do this with due reference to the healthcare system, best practice as commended in guidelines (e.g., NICE – National Institute for Health and Care Excellence), research evidence and care protocol.

Book structure

The book is arranged in two parts. The first part outlines the theory of person-centred care and a pragmatic interpretation of that in practice. In Chapter 1, I outline how notions of person-centred care have developed over time and how the professional origins of person-centred care have shaped those notions. While person-centred care has always been focussed on the wellbeing of patients, it has also served a purpose in defining and building the reputation of nursing (Butts and Rich, 2014). Where person-centred care is only presented in idealistic terms, however, it may lay itself open to a charge that it is unrealistic. So Chapter 1 is about conceptions of person-centred care, of service and it explores a problem.

In Chapter 2, I argue for a more pragmatic person-centred care, one that works better within care settings and the resources available there. My suggestions still centre on understanding patient perceptions of their illness and healthcare experiences. Decades ago Oermann and colleagues (Oermann et al., 1983) highlighted the importance of understanding patient perceptions. In a discussion of tracheostomy care they highlighted how the nurse's explanation of tube care mismatched with the patient's needs. The nurse explained the technical and procedural steps that she would use and the rationale for tube suction. The patient was instead concerned with how this might feel.

The second and largest part of this book is then divided into a series of chapters relating to different circumstances in which person-centred care might be re-examined. Each of the chapters is supported by a case study that enables you to explore person-centred care ideas. What is required to ensure that anxiety is managed or that the patients can rehabilitate well, for example? Case studies have purposefully been offered from different fields of practice. Each represents a new opportunity to demonstrate respect and support. The case studies are drawn from my clinical and consultancy work over the years and they function as teaching tools to illustrate how patients think and how nurses work. Narratives have been presented in ways that enable you to explore person-centred care themes.

The first chapters of Part 2 start with opening care relationships. I begin with establishing a rapport. A relationship has to begin and, in some circumstances, that has to happen very quickly indeed. Later the relationship develops and it might be tested in different ways. Perhaps treatment falters? Perhaps progress is not as fast as either the clinician or the patient hoped? As I move through the case-study chapters, I examine person-centred care within a context of new challenges. The chapters introduce you to ways in which evidence can be brought to bear as part of person-centred care. Part 2 of the book ends with a chapter looking forward to the future. How might nurses contribute their person-centred care insights to an improving service of the future?

Requirements for the NMC *Standards of Proficiency for Registered Nurses*

The Nursing and Midwifery Council (NMC) has established standards of proficiency to be met by applicants to different parts of the register, and these are the standards it considers necessary for safe and effective practice. This book is structured so that it will help you to understand and meet the proficiencies required for entry to the NMC register. The relevant proficiencies are presented at the start of each chapter so that you can clearly see which ones the chapter addresses. The proficiencies have been designed to be generic so that they apply to all fields of nursing and all care settings. This is because all nurses must be able to meet the needs of any person they encounter in their practice, regardless of their stage of life or health challenges, whether these are mental, physical, cognitive or behavioural.

This book includes the latest standards for 2018 onwards, taken from *Future Nurse: Standards of Proficiency for Registered Nurses* (NMC, 2018).

Learning features

Learning from reading text is not always easy. Therefore, to provide variety and to assist with the development of independent learning skills and the application of theory to practice, this book contains activities, case studies, further reading, useful websites and other materials to enable you to participate in your own learning. Please note that weblinks suggested within this book are live at the time the book goes to press. As the internet is a fast-changing environment some links may later change or be lost. Using key search terms such as person-centred care + the focus of interest (e.g., rehabilitation) should enable you to identity other relevant resources.

The activities in this book will help you to make sense of person-centred care in action. Some activities ask you to reflect on aspects of practice, or your experience of it, or the people or situations you encounter. *Reflection* is an essential skill in nursing, and it helps you to understand the world around you and often to identify how things might be improved. Other activities will help you develop key graduate skills such as your ability to *think critically* about a topic in order to challenge received wisdom. The book, in particular, illustrates how to combine an understanding of research evidence and patient narrative to recommend better care solutions. Communication and working as part of a team are core to all nursing practice, and some activities will ask you to think about your *communication skills* to help develop these abilities.

All the activities require you to take a break from reading the text, to think through the issues presented and to carry out some independent study, possibly using the internet. Where appropriate, there are sample answers presented at the end of each chapter and these will help you to understand more fully your own reflections and independent study. Remember, academic study will always require independent work; attending lectures will never be enough to be successful on your programme. These activities will help to deepen your knowledge and understanding of the issues under scrutiny and give you practice at working on your own.

You might want to think about completing these activities as part of your personal development plan (PDP) or portfolio. After completing the activity, write it up in your PDP or portfolio in a section devoted to that particular skill, then look back over time to see how far you are developing. You can also do more of the activities for a key skill in which you have identified a weakness, which will help build your skill and confidence in this area.

This book also contains a glossary on page 179 to assist you with unfamiliar terms. Glossary terms are in bold in the first instance that they appear.

Parting wish

Person-centred care is much more than an academic subject, a topic within the course. It is ultimately about what it feels like to nurse, about what can sustain you in a hopefully satisfying career within healthcare. Much of what sustains nurses is the feeling that they have been able to express their compassion for others in need. It is about feeling that you have made a tangible difference. I hope, then, that this text certainly assists you with your studies but that it will also enthuse you about what is possible in nursing. The book will certainly help with coursework and examinations, but it will also have worked best when it enhances your ongoing confidence to care. My best wishes for that, wherever you practise.

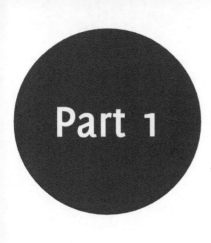

Part 1 Person-centred care

Theory and philosophy

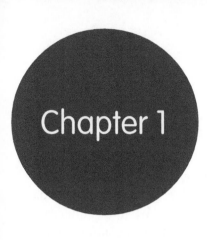

Chapter 1 · Person-centred care

Concepts, origins and problems

Chapter aims

After reading this chapter, you will be able to:

- understand the origins of person-centred care within nursing and how that can conflict with other notions of service to patients;
- understand why a tension is sometimes felt as regards how care should be delivered.

Introduction

If you were invited to decide whether you would prefer to deliver person-centred care or something more standardised, it would seem surprising if you elected the latter. We are taught to value people and how they cope with adversity. We are charged with protecting the vulnerable in our care. The NMC (2015) Code of Conduct (*The Code*) requires nurses to have proper regard for the needs and the experiences of the individual. We are challenged to find out what the patient's perceived needs are, what their goals may be, and to include these in a negotiation of care. We must understand patient feelings and preferences, as well as to consider care that is commended by research evidence, care protocols and policies, or the standards of bodies such as the National Institute for Health and Care Excellence (NICE) (Stanek, 2017).

Person-centred nursing care sounds an obviously good thing. To be person-centred is synonymous with understanding and helping patients (Doherty and Thompson, 2014; Sharp et al., 2016). It seems the ethical and the professional response to healthcare situations. In this chapter, however, I will explore the assumptions of person-centred care as described within the literature and highlight a number of concerns associated with that. That which seems ideal is not necessarily that which might yet be possible. At one extreme is idealised person-centred care where the emphasis is firmly on the individual and their perceived needs. At the other extreme is a service focussed on assured standards, policies and protocols for the many. Evolving ideas about consumerism fit between the two and may be claimed to be in support of both conceptions of care.

Understanding why there are different conceptions of care, between the **philosophical** and the **pragmatic**, is important if we are to care for patients with a due sense of pride in what is achieved. Finally, at the end of the chapter, I offer a working definition of person-centred care as it will be used in this textbook.

Activity 1.1 Reflecting

Pause now to consider what you think person-centred care actually entails. At this stage, don't worry if it is 'correct'. Jot your answers down so that you can return to them again as the explanations unfold within this chapter. To help guide you with this, consider the following questions:

1. How much choice can or should the patient be given in terms of treatment and care?
2. What do you assume as regards the patient's capabilities, their ability to collaborate in care?

3. Who in person-centred care has responsibilities for care work and outcomes?
4. What do you think is involved in getting to know the patient well enough to learn about their fears, needs and aspirations?

An outline answer is provided at the end of the chapter.

Key premises of person-centred care

Sharma et al. (2015) have reviewed the key premises (underpinning assumptions) of person-centred care as described within the literature.

1. That there is a **therapeutic relationship**. This means that a **rapport** has been established and that the patient feels confident in revealing their concerns, needs and hopes to the nurse. Equally, it means that the nurse feels able to explore and address patient concerns that extend beyond the usual treatment linked to a disease or illness. The nurse and the patient are cast as joint explorers of problem, need and preferred solution. In mental healthcare, for instance, Gabrielsson et al. (2014) describe the centrality of the therapeutic care relationship in helping patients to understand and confront the challenges of their illness.

2. That the patient and nurse share both power and responsibilities relating to care planned. Conventionally, patients exercise the power of informed consent. In some conceptions of person-centred care, however, patients choose courses of treatment and specify how they prefer to collaborate with healthcare professionals. Leplege et al. (2007), for example, highlight that the patient eventually becomes an **expert** on their illness. A well-educated and informed healthcare consumer may demand more than a less well-informed one, so ethical issues associated with resource allocation may become an issue. Partnership in care involves negotiation of expectations and responsibilities, yet expectations may sometimes be unrealistic (Tonnessen et al., 2017).

3. In person-centred care, the patient carries responsibility for their part in recovery or rehabilitation work. The patient is required to actively engage in care work with the nurse rather than to be a passive consumer of what clinicians recommend (e.g., McMahon et al., 2017). Culturally this may seem strange to some patients who have been more accustomed to a more passive patient role. It is not automatic that all patients wish to exercise additional power.

4. It is argued that the patient will become well known to the nurse as a person rather than simply as a patient (Doherty and Thompson, 2014). Establishing rapport with the patient requires significant skill on the part of the nurse (McCormack and McCance, 2017). He or she must be a skilled interviewer and be able to encourage the patient to ask questions, to make observations or requests.

Even though the care relationship often starts with more power for the nurse (because of their knowledge), the nurse works to shift the power base towards the patient by demonstrating that patient experience is equally important. Knowing the patient is not simply directed towards understanding them but to **empowering** them, so that they feel able to shoulder a greater share of decision-making responsibilities. Sharma et al. (2015) remind us that there are issues here, relating to:

- patient beliefs and values that might be deep-seated and not readily shared;
- assumptions about what counts as adequate health (wellbeing);
- different levels of health literacy (what the patient understands regarding illnesses and treatments); and
- preferences regarding how, when and where information is shared. A patient, for example, might expect the nurse to discuss their needs and concerns with a relative.

5. Communication within person-centred care must be regular, unrushed and often private. For trust and respect to develop the patient has to feel that they share information confidentially. The nurse will need to negotiate that which needs to be shared with other care team members, explaining the value of conferring with colleagues and making referrals in healthcare. As the care relationship develops, the nurse may have to act increasingly as a counsellor on choices, while ensuring that the final decision remains with the patient (Roberts, 2013).

As advocates of person-centred care, McCormack and McCance (2017) are keenly aware of the complexities of ideal person-centred care. They, for example, point out that we need to understand people in the context of their relationships with others such as the family. But the person, too, is assumed to be keenly self-aware. That is, they are reflective, introspective and have a considerable understanding of what matters most to them. This personal understanding of what motivates us and what our preferred role is, is what psychologists call **metacognition**. The patient knows his or her self extremely well.

It is in the context of these different ideas about people that McCormack and McCance (2017) introduce their framework for person-centred care. At the centre of care work is the person, their satisfaction with care, and what they hope to achieve as part of feeling well. Nurses need to create a 'therapeutic culture' that shifts the centre of healthcare work towards patient experience and need. Nurses work closely with the values and beliefs of the patient, understanding that not to do so means that change is unsustainable. A patient who does not believe in what has been recommended to them may be less likely to carry on with changes that are beneficial.

McCormack and McCance (2017) also acknowledge that for person-centred care to advance four things must be firmly in place.

1. Nurses must be emotionally and skill competent. They must have the necessary interpersonal skills, commitment, and clarity of beliefs and values associated with what seems most desirable in care activity. The nurse must have a good understanding of his or her self, expressing their values through care.

2. There must be a conducive care environment, one that accepts the necessity of shared decision making between clinicians and patients. There are significant implications here for the resourcing of the health service and role responsibilities when risk is assessed.

3. There must be person-centred care processes in place, the means by which agreed care can be planned and documented. The Gothenburg University Centre for Person-centred Care commissioned a series of research studies exploring what was involved in delivering person-centred care (Brittan et al., 2016). While there were similarities as regards the ethos of care, local practical measures were needed to accommodate the different care environments.

4. Expected outcomes had to be better explained. There are multiple ways in which person-centred care might be evaluated, for example in terms of expressed patient satisfaction, success in rehabilitation programmes, statistical improvements in body functions, and exercise tolerance. Without being clear about what is a claimed result of person-centred care, it is harder to persuade others to adopt it.

Activity 1.2   Critical thinking

Return now to the notes that you have made in response to the previous activity and then answer the following questions.

1. Has your understanding of person-centred care now expanded, involving additional insights into its complexity? If you think that your first understanding of person-centred care involved particular strengths or misconceptions, jot down what you think those were.
2. What do you now understand about commitment? The commitment of the nurse to fashion a new care relationship with the patient. The commitment required of a patient to think and act differently with the nurse. The commitment sought from healthcare organisations to change the way in which service is conceived.
3. What seems hopeful and what seems daunting about the conception of person-centred care as summarised above? Jot down what you think the issues are.

An outline answer is provided at the end of the chapter.

The above description of person-centred care may have encouraged you, but there are a number of reservations that should be recognised and these are summarised in Table 1.1.

Limitation	Notes
Undue optimism as regards availability of resources.	Highly individualised care planning with lots of patient choices presupposes generous resources, enough to address the competing demands of patients. A shift to pursuing the patient's goals, that which helped them to feel well, might deprive other patients of their perceived requirements. Resources of materials and nurses' time could quickly become overstretched. Patient–staff ratios would need to significantly improve.
Patients' expectations may increase and diversify ahead of whatever the health service did to respond to patient need.	Perceptions of need and of rights might rapidly change and escalate. In midwifery, for example, women sometimes argue that they have a right to caesarean sections even though vaginal delivery might carry fewer risks and confer benefits to babies. Patient felt need is not always superior to recommended clinical practice. Patients and clinicians may evaluate risk differently.
Idealised person-centred care assumes a significant degree of patient motivation, learning ability and willingness to self-care (Abotalebidariasari et al., 2016; Wazni and Gifford, 2017).	Curious, well-educated and motivated patients may be eager to take charge of their health once again, but not all patients are equally well-motivated or so confident.
Significant assumptions are made about the skill level of the nurse. The nurse is cast as therapist, counsellor, teacher, mentor (Sharp et al., 2016).	Nurses working within clinical nurse specialist or advanced practitioner roles already have these skills but they are not as widespread as nurse philosophers might hope. In acute care, where contact time is perhaps limited, there may be limited time to practice the required skills.
Personal and clinical care agendas are necessarily different.	The clinical agenda is often about managing risk and improving the efficacy of chosen treatments. The service must be efficient as well as effective. Personal agendas of the patient are often about experience and comfort.

Table 1.1 Limitations of idealised person-centred care

While accepting the above limitations, there would arguably also be some gains in adopting a person-centred care approach. Not only might levels of patient satisfaction with a service improve markedly, but there may be more successful use of treatments and rehabilitation services. That which the patient embraces, is that which the patient uses to best effect (Glass et al., 2012).

In 1951 the sociologist Talcott Parsons described what he called the 'sick role' and explained that it had both rights and responsibilities attached. The patient had a right to be excused from their normal life responsibilities, precisely because they were ill. They had a right to expect help from healthcare professionals. But their responsibilities included sincerely wishing to get better and to take up once again the responsibilities of healthy citizens. It is critical today to renew that clear sense of rights and responsibilities for patients at a time when the diversity of treatment has exploded and care is delivered in many different locations. The more we can articulate what patients as well as clinicians are expected to do, the easier it may be to advance the quality of healthcare.

While person-centred care presumes a significant increase in the skill level of clinicians, that in itself might prove professionally satisfying and motivating. In midwifery, for example, the birth plan offers the woman considerable choice, and that might then be modified as risks arise and parties discuss what seems an acceptable way forward (Way and Scammell, 2016). Midwives are able to deploy their skills, advising an anxious but otherwise healthy mother-to-be why a caesarean section might not be the wise default option for the forthcoming birth.

Person-centred care certainly has the potential to effect significant improvements in patient care. Patients may feel more respected, consulted with, better supported and more confident to carry on improving their health when the care relationship has concluded. Notions such as that of therapeutic use of self in mental health nursing assume that nurses will work closely with the patient, using their own life experiences to help patients solve problems (Gabrielsson et al., 2014). Within the field of intellectual disabilities, it is vital that the nurse understands how the service user habitually learns (Codling, 2015). What remains complicated is that person-centred care is conceived of slightly differently in different care environments. Therefore, considerable work remains to be done on the expression of person-centred care in different settings.

Activity 1.3 Practice reviewing

Take a moment now to write down one practice from your place of work or a clinical placement where you have identified care shifting to focus on patient **felt needs**. Did this rely on what the current patient told you or did it draw on what an accumulation of patient experience offered? What are the benefits, then, of listening to patients and learning about how they perceive the care that is delivered?

An outline answer is provided at the end of the chapter.

The origins of person-centred care and competing philosophies

Having introduced person-centred care's key premises, it is now time to briefly examine where this philosophy and its competitors started from. This is not merely an academic exercise, but something that helps to explain some of the difficulties that you may have when trying to practise in a person-centred way. For you to sustain practice over many decades it is important that you feel that what you do is coherent with your care philosophy. Each day that you go to work you test care, to see what seems personally satisfying, effective, efficient and of the highest quality.

Ohlen et al. (2017) describe the tensions that arise when philosophers arguing for a healthcare centred strongly on the individual clash with those arguing for one that centres on 'good service' for the public. When philosophers propose a certain course, describe the history of their ideas in their preferred terms, this is called a **discourse**. It discusses what is happening and frequently includes beliefs about what they think should happen next. When other competing discourses are offered up, arguments arise about which is best. So advocates of person-centred care clash with those who advocate for group needs and a greater standardisation of care. Both claim to have at their centre a concern for people and their wellbeing, but each differs as regards the right way to serve the public. The person-centred care philosopher might observe that the others' view of care is bureaucratic, insensitive and sometimes even inhumane. The service philosopher might counter claim that the others' view of care is naïve, idealistic, open to service fragmentation and difficult to develop as part of evidence-based practice.

In healthcare today there are three discourses describing healthcare and the proper focus of nurses.

1. Person-centred care (with a greater focus on the individual – it is argued that health, and more especially wellbeing, is understood at the individual level and it is there that we should focus our work).

2. Group-centred care (this tends to emphasise the importance of standardising care, so that everyone has the clearest possible idea of what a service has to offer).

3. **Consumer-led care.** This is a relatively new discourse and it emphasises the critical ability of individuals or groups of people to evaluate needs and preferences, and to use and judge services. The growth of the internet with its health and illness information has fuelled consumerism (Shrank, 2017). Both of the preceding discourses on healthcare appeal to thinkers in this camp. Person-centred care philosophers argue that consumerism highlights the growing confidence of patients to negotiate their own care. Group-centred, quality assurance philosophers emphasise the need for a care package to be distinct, clear and well-reasoned, so the consumer knows to what he or she has contracted.

Activity 1.4   Reflecting

Try to think now of examples of care from your experience (either as a patient or a nurse) that you think were strongly influenced by person-centred, group-centred and consumer-centred care thinking. What do you think was commendable in each case? Does what we call 'quality care' differ markedly depending on which approach to care you adopt?

An outline answer is provided at the end of the chapter.

The person-centred care discourse

Olsson and Ung (2012) explain that person-centred care has its origins within the holistic care movement of the 1960s. **Holism** argues that human beings are more than the sum of their parts. People have physical, psychological, social and spiritual needs. It is the interplay of these, and how these are managed in a life context, that defines what it is to be human. In the 1970s and 1980s much of the nursing literature was shaped by arguments relating to holistic care. That is, nurses were meant to ascertain all the relevant needs of patients, relating to an illness or injury event, within the physical, the social, psychological and spiritual domains. One of the problems with the holism argument was that it was sometimes difficult to demonstrate something from each of the domains within the care plan, simply as a matter of form. Not all of the domains were equally relevant in care situations, but nurses were sometimes pressed to include them as part of work to ensure that patients weren't simply treated as physical bodies ('the wound in bed 9').

The enthusiastic adoption of holistic care thinking within nursing needs to be understood in the context of political changes underway within the healthcare professions. In the 1960s, textbooks for nurses were still called 'medical nursing' or 'surgical nursing'. Nursing care was seen as a supplement to the medical intervention and usually as subservient to the physician-directed one at that. During the same period, however, nurse theorists introduced the 'nursing process', insisting that nurses made their own independent assessment of patient needs, which complemented the medical assessment of treatment requirements. If doctors focussed on the body and perhaps on particular parts of it, then nurses focussed on the person and their experiences (Brooker and Waugh, 2013).

Person-centred care built on the principles of holistic care and argued for the importance of nurse input into the definition of care and of excellence. It is not surprising that person-centred care focused so sharply upon the nurse–patient relationship for this was a means of protecting the distinctive contribution of nursing to the health service. Having cast off the dominance of the medical profession though, nursing had then been confronted with a new threat, the reconceptualisation of healthcare as a managed service, one that was no longer dominated by professions but that was increasingly rationalised and run as a public sector business (Gabe and Calnan, 2009).

So, the discourse of person-centred care not only attends to the rights and needs of individuals, something latterly wholeheartedly taken up by the World Health Organisation (McCormack and McCance, 2017), but it attended as well to the political agenda of nursing. To protect nursing within an increasingly difficult healthcare environment it was critical to emphasise the increasing expertise and skills of nurses. If healthcare was to be improved, then it was (argued to be) important that the patient experienced elements of care, and their interpretation of improvement was emphasised as much as treatment outcomes. Pressing an ever greater emphasis on care as a process, rather than as a standardised service, meant that there remained scope for nurses to use their skills to fashion care solutions that seemed important to nurses as well as beneficial to patients (Rankin, 2015). Care as a negotiated process also helped to counter what was perceived as **managerialism**. This involved extending claims regarding the traditional remit of past nursing practice. However, the difficulties of enacting this remained. It was difficult to demonstrate how nursing care served wide-ranging areas of wellbeing. It was difficult to argue for resources that would allow nurses to extend their roles, becoming consultants in care, unless clear resource utilisation priority outcomes could be demonstrated.

The group-centred quality assurance discourse

The group-centred quality assurance discourse has its origins in the inception of the British National Health Service (NHS). Prior to 1948, care services were fragmented and dependent to a large extent on individual hospitals, insurance schemes and charitable organisations. Much greater control was exercised by medicine both in primary and secondary care. Following the deprivations of the 1920s and 1930s and two world wars however, the new NHS was conceived of as a cradle-to-grave service that removed many of the worries of British citizens (Rivett, 1998). The emphasis was on service and on a completeness and coherence of provision. Within the new system practitioners from different professions would work together to improve the coverage of assistance offered and to ensure that service was as seamless as possible. What is sometimes under-emphasised is that the new service emphasised co-ordinated work (Gorsky, 2013). It was not a system designed to promote the territory interests of different professions, although throughout its history the NHS has been a place of both professional co-operation and rivalry.

Plans to provide a cradle-to-grave service were tested during subsequent decades. It became harder to promise a universal provision. Nonetheless, the success of the NHS was significant, reducing the levels of mortality and morbidity within the British population and with little or no point-of-access cost to patients (Welch, 2018). As patients

- lived longer,
- dealt with more chronic illnesses relating to ageing and lifestyle,
- and as professions learned to treat and manage more conditions,

so the demands on the NHS grew exponentially.

From the 1980s onwards, governments began to remodel the healthcare service so that quality care was still maintained but the organisation worked more efficiently (Gorsky, 2013). The costs of the NHS, left within clinician hands, were seen to be increasing rapidly and it was now necessary to rationalise care services. The designers of the NHS had hoped that timely treatment would incrementally reduce subsequent need. In practice, however, the more the NHS provided, the more the public demanded of it. More and more treatments, procedures and services were added to the remit. The introduction of general managers, those charged with costing, prioritising and rationing services, would assist politicians in sustaining their promises on issues such as patient waiting times.

The remodelling of healthcare as a business, one that was not only effective but also cost efficient, came as a challenge to the healthcare professions (Traynor, 1999; Cope et al., 2015). Each profession had been growing its sphere of influence, arguing for the importance of its work. Now, in the face of efficiency agendas, nursing was faced with uncomfortable decisions. Traditional care came under threat. Some nurses argued that they might do medical work more cost-effectively. Duties moved from doctors to nurses and from nurses to care assistants. But other nurses lamented that the traditional remit of nursing was being lost in the pursuit of changing roles. So, just as the discourse of group need and assured quality care moved to efficiency as well as effectiveness debates, nurses re-emphasised that to which doctors or others could not so readily attend. Helping patients to make sense of their needs, to cope with illness (something more personal than disease), became the increasing focus of nursing philosophy (Traynor, 1999). The group-care discourse in contrast had always acknowledged the need for flexible workers, teams and services that were coherent and fit for purpose. However, that discourse now centred on increasingly defined standards and outputs. The work of the team and, beyond that, of the service, was deemed of greater importance than that of any single profession.

The patient–consumer discourse

The patient–consumer discourse had its greatest momentum from the late 1980s when a series of government white papers, such as *Working for Patients* (Department of Health, 1989a) and *Caring for People: Community Care in the Next Decade and Beyond* (Department of Health, 1989b), described patients in consumerist terms. Before then, patient advocacy organisations arguing for a greater voice in healthcare provision had begun, but the emphasis was not on the individual consumer (Mold, 2015).

From the 1990s successive British governments used the concerns of patients as consumers to press for healthcare re-organisation agendas (Harrison and McDonald, 2007). The status of healthcare trusts was to be enhanced with representation by patients on governing and advisor panels, and the primary care organisations' commissioning services were required to find a means of securing patient–consumer opinion on what was needed and what worked best.

The notion of patients as individual consumers grew alongside the healthcare organisational changes and with close reference to several influential developments:

- the growth and diversification of sources of patient information, most notably on the internet (Morgan, 2016);
- the improved organisation of charities supporting patients with particular agendas and needs;
- The mass media politicisation of healthcare service debates, disputes and shortfalls.

Media exposure of care deficits encouraged patients to become more discriminating in their assessment and selection of services. Brown et al. (2011) explained that, as a result, the public became increasingly sceptical of both professional and managerial claims relating to health, treatment and care.

However, Mold (2015) reminds us that patient consumerism was always in some degree problematic. Patients (in Britain) did not directly purchase care, unlike those in other countries using a medical insurance or a pay-at-point-of-care system. The leverage of the patient was more modest within a welfare state healthcare system. Patient consumerism was hampered by:

- significant asymmetry between knowledge held by the contracting parties – while patients had more information through the internet, this was not as coherent as that gleaned from a professional training, from research or audit of service (Calnan, 2010);
- patients often contracted care during periods of stress – the shift from care founded on clinician-identified need, to patient goal, from that which was essential to that which seemed optimal in the consumer's view, was always going to be challenging (Newman and Vidler, 2006);
- patient expertise took time to develop – while a patient dealing over the course of years with a health deficit would develop expertise, this was sometimes arduous learning.

Today, the patient as consumer discourse remains vibrant, but it is also fragmented. Patients are not a homogenous group and those with particular needs turn to advocates who can fight their cause. While there may be concerted calls for better and clearer information, the setting out of treatment options within what is affordable (for instance by NICE guidelines) and for more considerate handling of questions and suggestions by patients, the discourse focusses as much upon enough service and clear service as upon how it is best delivered. While both advocates of person-centred care and group-centred care might beckon the consumer to their cause, a degree of cynicism about professional recommendation on both sides may make the consumer a difficult ally to secure. Table 1.2 summarises the competing claims and limits of the discourses outlined here.

	Person-centred care	Consumer-focussed care	Group-centred care
Care focus	The individual and their relatives.	Proactive members of the public, inquisitive and discerning as regards healthcare service.	Populations of patients at large, those that experience common difficulties and needs.
Premises	That the patient actively engages in healthcare issues and is confident to do so. That the nurse is skilled and confident to explore a range of concerns and needs with the patient beyond that immediately linked to disease, injury or treatment.	That individuals are confident in researching needs and services, the better to articulate their expectations of care. Individuals may contract care with others working on their behalf (for instance, charity-linked groups who represent recurring concerns and needs).	That people respect that care is a finite resource to be shared, and that it is better that the priority needs of the many require the earliest and greatest attention of the healthcare professional. The duty of the service is to articulate the offer clearly and to ensure that it is consistently, rigorously and safely delivered.

Strengths	Care seems liberal and individually articulated. It provides increasing choice, that which attends to what it means to feel and be well.	Care reflects the needs articulated by groups of individuals who understand particular healthcare problems met with in common.	Minimum care standards are sustained through the better articulation of what the service provides. The public understands the limits of a contracted service, that arranged through government and its agencies.
Limitations	Significant resource limitations impinge on what the nurse can contract individually with patients. Patients and nurses may be unready for the shared care negotiation that the philosophy espouses. Boundaries of care negotiation may become tested, for instance, patients may not wish to discuss some intimate areas of healthcare need.	Better represented consumer groups may secure a growing share of the total care resource. Patient consumer groups may openly compete with one another to determine the nature of service. The expertise of healthcare professionals may be challenged as felt need competes with research-recommended practice.	The care service seems less than ideal, meeting some priority demands but ignoring many other felt needs. The service seems increasingly insensitive and bureaucratic, rating issues relating to efficiency above those of effectiveness or humanity.
Implications for nurses	The nurse must become a skilled negotiator and a facilitator of strategies designed to meet mutually agreed goals. Traditional notions of nursing work centred on disease or injury, shift to illness experience and work onwards to health and wellbeing. The diversity of nursing work increases.	Nurses and others must mediate competing demands for the resources available. The nurse becomes someone who liaises with consumer groups to better articulate the most important services. Nurses advise consumers on sources of information, recommending some and countering others, using their own knowledge of evidence.	Nurses operate consistently within protocols and policies, those designed to protect the patient but also to manage service budgets. Nurses have to explain the limits of the service available, but also to point patients to other resources that they might pursue.

Table 1.2   Competing discourses on how care should be arranged

Activity 1.5   Critical thinking

With a colleague, identify why the three different discourses on healthcare complicate what the nurse is asked to do in the support of patients. The following summaries may help.

(Continued)

(Continued)

- Person-centred care offers the patient more choice and more influence, but it also assigns them responsibilities that could seem challenging. To make choices patients might be asked to share more personal information, the better to determine needs, preferences and goals.
- Group-centred care assures the patient of packages of care and minimum standards associated with their operation, treatment or rehabilitation, but, beyond respectful attention to them as a client, it might fail to identify individual worries and needs.
- The patient–consumer discourse highlights the searching of patients for information and service that best suits their objectives. Consumers might become increasingly sophisticated, but the confidence to insist on requirements might not always be founded on the most complete or most authoritative information.

An outline answer is provided at the end of the chapter.

A pragmatic person-centred care definition

Your discussions in response to Activity 1.5 may well have led you to conclude that the issue of care arrangement remains rather confused. Whatever you thought person-centred care compromised of (Activity 1.1), it might now seem a little more complicated. Whatever you thought of standard care pathways in practice, it is now clearer why there was a search for something that could be assured to everyone. Both the needs of the individual and of the wider group remains a balance to be struck during each shift that the nurse completes. Patients as consumers may become more exacting, and the nurse is drawn into discussions of what seems wise as well as what seems desirable. Some of what shapes a good care outcome stems from the sensitive understanding of the patient's circumstances, needs and personal ways of coping. Some of what constitutes good care comes from the appliance of research evidence, lessons learned from the experience of work with many patients, from knowledge relating to pharmacy, physiology, wound healing, child development, mental illness, ageing processes and a range of other empirical information.

Care is less of a mess than we might think, however. While nurses and others have views on how care should be delivered, clinicians often agree reasonable compromises with patients (Elwyn et al., 2016). Patients are amenable to well-explained research evidence and they are welcoming of the clinician's assessment of risk attendant on different courses of action. Consumers may press a cause, but there is a widespread recognition that goals might have to be met in concert with different people and using different avenues. Without reference to a particular philosophy, clinicians incrementally notice what concerns a particular group of patients as needful most often and start there. They learn to read what patients want to understand first, given the environment in which they find themselves. Local groups of clinicians, nurses and others begin to innovate, asking questions about what would make care and support better for the patient. That might attend to a number of things, for example who works first with the patient, who explains particular things, how information is shared, and how options are explored. What characterises those working environments is that they are communication-rich, across the group of professionals collaborating and with the patients and lay carers involved.

In practice, there is often no pure ideological care approach in action. 'Person-centred care' offers some well-developed off-the-peg solutions that are adapted to suit patient-expressed need. Group-centred care includes aide memoires by which nurses check the experience of the patient, ascertaining what seems uncomfortable or unsuccessful. Clinicians appreciate that not all that can be done is necessarily supplied by healthcare professionals. There may be additional support that can be recommended elsewhere. We will be exploring a theory of such pragmatism in the next chapter. For now, however, it is important to offer a definition of person-centred care as it will be used in this textbook. It is one that acknowledges a compromise between the needs of the individual and of the many, one that opens up opportunities for patients and that commends the expertise of the nurse. It is a definition directed to helping patients to feel respected, consulted, sometimes challenged, always valued, but necessarily the clients of a service too.

Person-centred nursing care (pragmatic)

Person-centred care is a relationship developed with a patient that demonstrates due regard for their personal experience and perceptions of the current situation, which enables them to feel respected, supported and valued during healthcare. It assists the patient to take stock of their circumstances and to explore options for the future, options that may be dependent on what the patient does as well as what is offered as part of service. Person-centred care assures the person that we have regard for their wellbeing, a life that has personal meaning, but it also insists on the nurse's roles as consultant, expert and advisor, roles that involve sharing evidence, experience and best practice wisdom. Person-centred care is facilitative; it enables the patient to engage and debate to the extent that they feel comfortable, and it always acknowledges their right to informed consent, to accept, augment, to change, to refuse, courses of action, while also accepting their personal responsibility for the decisions they make.

Chapter summary

This chapter has explained what person-centred care is, as expressed within the literature, and has summarised the ways in which the history of ideas within healthcare have shaped arguments surrounding this concept. While person-centred care sounds

(Continued)

(Continued)

deceptively simple, it becomes rather more complex when it is set out within institutional settings and where multiple expectations of care are expressed. Person-centred care becomes a focus for those arguing about the rightful place of nursing, and for developing ideas about service and better responses to what consumers might expect of healthcare professionals.

- Person-centred care might be conceived in more or less idealistic terms, those that make assumptions about the resources available and the skills of the nurse. At one extreme is a person-centred care that transforms the whole of healthcare and centres on far-reaching and very individual care negotiation. At the other extreme (the pragmatic) is a person-centred care that humanises healthcare systems, which preserves and supports the dignity of patients.
- Much care, however, remains focussed on service to the many, a consistent minimum standard that all can expect. This understanding of care centres on assurances about service, rather than extensive assurances about the freedom to negotiate care.
- Because the nurse is encouraged to think of person-centred care as part of nursing philosophy as well as of service, there is a risk that nurses find it harder to know how best to proceed in particular circumstances. Artful compromises have to be found between theory and practice, between idealism and pragmatism and that is the subject of the remainder of this book.

Activities: Brief outline answers

Activity 1.1 Reflecting (pp8–9)

You may have thought of person-centred care as an attitude, a way of thinking of the patient as a person rather than simply as someone who enacts a role. If so, excellent! That is the essence of person-centred care, understanding the person who finds themselves in the role of the patient, their fears and worries, their perceived needs and goals. But, once we move into what that practically entails, some complications arise. The choice afforded patients depends not only on the resources available within the health service, but the readiness and the ability of the patient to make choices. Without the relevant and accurate information, and a readiness to critically evaluate that information, it is much harder for the patient to make sound decisions. Depending on where you work and the placements that you have completed, you may have noted that patients varied widely in their capabilities to make choices regarding care. Some patients might even insist that they don't want the responsibility of making lots of choices, that they think of that as the professional's responsibility. One of the recurring problems in healthcare is that it takes time to get to know patients sufficiently well to engage them as partners in care decision making. We need to understand, for example, how they think about risk; are they risk adverse or risk embracing?

Activity 1.2 Critical thinking (p11)

Your response to this activity is necessarily very personal but I offer a reflection on the matter of commitment (question 2). If we presume for a moment that in person-centred care the patient becomes our partner in care planning, delivery and evaluation, then that involves rights and responsibilities. To insist on patient rights without also acknowledging patient responsibilities leaves the nurse in the invidious position of directing less in care but remaining responsible for all care outcomes. Commitment, then, is required of both nurses and patients. Whether a passage of care is person-centred may be determined not only by what the nurse facilitates or contributes, but also by what the patient allows or offers as well. As we shall see in Part 2 of this book, patients vary widely in their capacity and readiness to engage with the nurse in the care process. The nurse rightly encourages and facilitates person-centred care, but success may depend on finding the best ways to help patients both expect more of and contribute more to care.

Activity 1.3   Practice reviewing (p13)

Listening to and learning from patients offers a wide range of benefits. Some that I thought of included learning about how patients solve problems and learning how they signal when they are worried or in pain. Listening to patients acquaints us with their other support resources, the lay carers that we might successfully liaise with. Some patients become an expert on their illness and may acquaint us with more successful ways of managing diet, medication or exercise.

Activity 1.4   Reflecting (p14)

Person-centred care examples are presented in the case studies of Part 2 of this book, but it is worth noting from the outset that these vary quite widely from quite discrete ways of talking with a patient to a shift in the way that care is delivered. In Chapter 3, for example, the nurse listens to the patient's worries in a particular way. In Chapter 5, patient education is designed in a different way. Group-centred care is often evidenced in particular programmes of support, those linked to a disease and in common rehabilitation problems. A patient education video, for example, is designed assuming some common needs on the part of patients. Quality is defined in different ways. For example, it might be judged with regard to flexibility, the extent to which the patient can shape what is done. Quality too, though, might be judged with reference to the extent to which things are explained and the coverage of patient guidance. The first emphasises care as process, the second emphasises care as product.

Activity 1.5   Critical thinking (pp19–20)

Here are three reasons why I think that the competing discourses could complicate care.

1. They set up different expectations of care among patients. Depending on what the patient has read or heard from others, patients may expect different things of nurses. The role of patient (as a consumer, as a partner, as a user of healthcare products) has changed in ways that it is harder for the nurse to anticipate.

2. Patients may discover that nurses have radically different expectations of them. For example, a nurse who assumes that the patient will enthusiastically engage in shared decision making may wonder about the motivation of a patient who had expected to play a more passive role.

3. Debates might ensue as regards the place of lay care, i.e., that provided by relatives. If the nurse understands more about the patient as a person, then that raises issues about the expertise of the lay carer. What does he or she contribute if not knowledge about the patient as a person?

Further reading

While Chapter 1 references a number of different person-centred care philosophy books, all of which might be explored with benefit, you might find a couple of applied person-centred care textbooks especially illuminating.

Marshall, M and Gilliard, J (2014) *Creating Culturally Appropriate Outside Spaces and Experiences for People With Dementia.* London: Jessica Kingsley Publishers.

Nothing attacks our sense of self more than dementia. That which we accumulated in memories in relationships is relentlessly eroded. This collection of essays, from different parts of the world, describes initiatives to help preserve the sense of person and of dignity of people suffering from dementia and I think it is quite uplifting.

Koubel, G and Bungay, H (2009) *The Challenge of Person-Centred Care: An Interprofessional Perspective.* Basingstoke: Palgrave Macmillan.

This collection of essays looks at person-centred care from a variety of different professional perspectives and it argues that unless the service from all is joined up, the experience of care is at best inconsistent.

Useful websites

The following sources all enable you to read further on the definitions of person-centred care and to capture some of the debates about what is entailed in delivering it. Importantly, the documents speak to the public at large. They are not directed specifically at nurses.

https://healthinnovationnetwork.com/.../what_is_person-centred_care-and_why_is_it_ important?

Health Innovation Network South London (accessed April 2018, no date for document declared).

https://valuingpeople.org.au/the-resource/what-is-person-centred-care

Valuing People. What is person-centred care?

www.health.org.uk/sites/health/files/HelpingMeasurePersonCentredCare.pdf

The Health Foundation: Inspiring Improvement, de Silva, D (2014) Helping measure person-centred care. Evidence review, March.

Chapter 2 A pragmatic approach to person-centred care

Chapter aims

After reading this chapter, you will be able to:

* understand the features of an approach to person-centred care that is realisable within the resources of a healthcare service;
* understand that the approach centres on different sorts of work that the nurse (and others) engage in.

Introduction

A pragmatic approach to person-centred care is more than the expression of good professional manners. It is more than simply listening to what patients have to tell us. It does involve a reconsideration of how care is arranged. But it is, too, something that relies on the imagination of local care givers and care recipients, an identification of what seems to work well, what seems reassuring and encouraging. In this sense a pragmatic expression of person-centred care is much less reliant on a grand theory and much more open to local discoveries. Instead of expressing the design of person-centred care in prescriptive terms, practitioners strive for solutions that have local appeal. Importantly, both patients and practitioners must like what is done. It must seem satisfying, purposeful and replicable over time as well as meeting professional care standards (e.g., Riding et al., 2017; Rose and Yates, 2015).

With this in mind, this chapter on the pragmatic design of person-centred care is not something that introduces a complex theory. Instead, it characterises some features of person-centred care that seem realisable. Importantly, it highlights how person-centred care can operate in process. One of the criticisms of some nurse-philosopher-conceived person-centred care is that it is unduly complex. A more pragmatic conception of person-centred care accepts that the person is centre stage, but it insists, too, that a range of healthcare personnel and services might work with the patient to effect satisfying solutions to care problems (Wigert and Wikstrom, 2014). Person-centred care is a collaborative tool, one that helps make care seamless, as well as one that celebrates what the nurse contributes.

In this chapter, person-centred care is described in terms of five elements of work. The work elements are presented as part of a developing support relationship between the patient and the service. Attention to each element of work increases the chances that the patient will feel that their care has been individual. Importantly, it will have helped to shift the perceived role of patients, encouraging them to become active participants in care. If patients are to achieve their personal goals of recovery and rehabilitation, there is usually some element of personal work required (Bigi, 2014). That which achieves and sustains a sense of wellbeing requires personal commitment. In a classic sociological study of how lay carers evaluate healthcare services, Baruch (1981) noted that, initially, services were often positively evaluated. As time went on, however, and lay carers paused to consider whether patients had achieved the goals that they set for themselves, the evaluation of service deteriorated (he referred to these as 'atrocity stories'). Service users tended to evaluate support and care more negatively as time went by. The paradox was that goal achievement often relied on patient/lay carer contributions too. It was less than honest to evaluate the failure to secure goals solely in terms of perceived professional support shortfalls.

While it is true that some patients have limited capacity to self-care and to partner staff in care work, others have potential to do more. This seems a vital shift if, over the longer term, service is to work more strategically with an ageing population of patients and with many who live with chronic illness. The move from 'being sick' to 'living well' necessarily involves learning and some share of responsibility for patients (Schopf et al., 2015).

Activity 2.1 Critical thinking

Are there any advantages in seeing person-centred care as involving different sorts of work? How does that differ from, say, conceiving of it in terms of ideals, standards or tasks completed for the patient? Nurses go to work, it implies a conscious application of ideas, of experience and insights, but do we always work by thinking hard about why we practice in particular ways?

An outline answer is provided at the end of the chapter.

Anticipating concerns, needs and requirements

While it would be tempting to imagine person-centred care starting with questions put to the new patient, here it is argued that the work starts well before that encounter. Nurses and other healthcare practitioners need to conduct serious preparatory work associated with their care environment (Stirk and Sanderson, 2012). Staff need to anticipate and articulate the concerns, needs and requirements that patients typically have when they come into their care. While there is no single archetype patient, it is arguable that most patients will have several common concerns and needs associated with the healthcare change that the service mediates. It is in anticipating the concerns, needs and requirements of patients that evidence, that from research, audit and clinical experience, is important.

Activity 2.2 Practice reviewing

Pause now to list the concerns, needs and requirements that you think that the patients you care for commonly share. These may be closely associated with illnesses that you help them to tackle, but it may also relate to therapies, operations or procedures that you use. They may also refer to the patient history that the individual brings to the healthcare setting.

Next, jot down a note about how you got this information. How do you know what you do about patients' concerns, needs and requirements?

As this answer is based on your own observation, there is no outline answer at the end of the chapter.

It is quite likely that within your care setting you care for more than one group of patients and that each of those groups might have a cluster of shared concerns, needs and requirements. Concerns relate to worries or uncertainty about what the health change may involve. Concerns relate to what the change signifies and what might be involved in future lifestyle. Needs may relate to getting through the change as safely as possible. Needs are about the adjustments necessary. Requirements are issues to do with being adequately equipped to play a confident part in that change. So, for example, a person learning to be an ostomist requires stoma care skills (Lim et al., 2015). On a cancer care ward, patients may complete different cancer drug regimens. But what they have in common is in coming to terms with the idea that they are using medications that have varying levels of side effects. The patients are coping with the ambiguous nature of treatment (Weeks et al., 2012). In a mental healthcare environment, patients might be dealing with subtly different diagnoses, but what they often have in common is that they share some form of group therapy (Lorentzen and Ruud, 2014).

Understanding the commonly felt concerns, needs and requirements is a prerequisite to person-centred care for several reasons.

- Unless we understand the commonly recurring experiences of patients, we are unlikely to seem assured about our ability to help the next patient. This is critical to the first rapport that we try to build with the patient. Trust is founded upon perceived expertise (e.g., Schaepe and Ewers, 2017). *We must sound as though we know what we are talking about,* for it is what we say we are doing and why that reassures the patient that we understand the change that they are going through.
- Anything that we ask the patient to do, for example self-administering insulin, dealing with a panic attack, countering voices heard in the head, is more likely to succeed if we have clarified typically what patients find easy or difficult, and what they manage to do with some degree of success (e.g., Klinke et al., 2013). In showing that we knew and understood other patients, we convey to the new patients that we have considerable regard for patient experience.
- Understanding the commonly experienced concerns, needs and requirements of care in our area of care narrows down that which has to be negotiated individually with the patient. For sure, the patient that we care for next may be quite different, but, statistically, patients share quite a lot in common. The act of taking stock of common patient-felt concerns, needs and requirements enables us to target our enquiries with a patient, when time may be limited and resources finite. Perti et al. (2014), for example, profile the risks of fatigue associated with cancer chemotherapy.
- Understanding commonly felt patient concerns, needs and requirements may enable us to question therapies, treatments or practices that, however clinically valuable, are not well received by patients. An effective treatment must work, it must be cost efficient to use and, critically, it must be acceptable to the patient. The more we have anticipated how treatments and care measures might be received, the more strategically we can recommend solutions.

One of the problems that nurses face when planning to deliver person-centred care is that the team of which they are a part has not studied common patient experiences and needs in advance. The team may have assumed that they know what seems most important to the patient. This means that there is less coherent 'good practice' knowledge to use as the basis for questions posed to the patient and the first assurances given to them and their relatives. Patients may become anxious if staff concerns seem to spread in many different directions; if their enquiries of patients are widely divergent. That which assures is that which seems both focussed (they understand issues) and that which is experienced by me, the patient (it is relevant).

Information from past patients can be obtained in a number of different ways. These include:

- patient experience of service audits, that which is sometimes added as commentary to satisfaction questionnaires;
- case studies, especially those that have been studied that are associated with risk-management procedures;
- patients' letters of complaint and of congratulation – letters of congratulation are most valuable where they explain why something seemed so good;
- research studies conducted both locally and elsewhere with patients undergoing similar healthcare changes (qualitative data research is especially important here);
- student nurse feedback – this might surprise you but the student brings to practice placements a fresh understanding and, because of their concerns to relate well to patients, they attend closely to what patients say.

Activity 2.3   Reflecting

Think about clinical placements that you have completed or places where you have worked. What were you briefed upon as regards the patient experience when you joined the team? Where you received such a briefing, where did the staff obtain their information? Have you shared your insights regarding the patient experience with qualified staff? If so, what did you hope they might do with that feedback?

For future placement planning, identify a patient concern that you suspect could be important to patients that you will nurse there. Plan how you will record in your placement portfolio/notes what you notice about that concern. Alert staff of your interest in this topic at first meeting to better plan how your insights might assist the team in their future work.

An outline answer is provided at the end of the chapter.

Hearing the patient narrative

The second sort of work relates to how human beings narrate their experiences to themselves and others, the better to make sense of what happens (Rosa, 2014). We are story-telling people. If you pause to consider your life to date, it is highly likely that what seemed especially eventful, what seemed valuable or daunting, has been interpreted using stories, some of which you have repeated and adjusted over time. *Do you remember the day that we … ?*

The psychological need to narrate experience rests with the ambiguity of events that we interpret. A range of stimuli (visual, auditory, tactile, olfactory) reach us quickly and, if memory does not offer an easy template to explain what is happening, we need to process the experience by trying out explanations (Taipale, 2014). What we think is happening, what that represents as a threat, a comfort, a challenge or reward, is every bit as powerful as reality itself. Perceptions have a significant effect on stress levels and our sense of wellbeing. Consider, for example, some of your earliest visits to the dentist. Irrespective of what an inspection of your mouth might reveal, the visit was quite probably already forming as a perceptual 'event' before you sat in the dentist's chair.

When nurses meet patients they need to establish what their perceptions of events are, and what their expectations of care and their relationship with the nurse might be (Price, 2017a). The reaching of a mutually agreeable perception of partnership, support and respect is part of the early work done by nurses when they meet patients. Of course not all patients are equally well placed to share their perceptions. Those that arrive with us in pain, semi-conscious, those affected by drugs or poisons or suffering a psychological crisis, for example, are not nearly so well placed to begin a negotiated care relationship.

Eliciting patient narratives is not always easy. Patients have to trust the nurse before they divulge a great deal about their experiences. There are, however, a number of measures that can help the patient to share their thoughts. These include the following.

- Ensuring that the patient has a safe place to talk. That explained in public settings may well be much more guarded.
- Explaining at the outset how we will use information and where it will be shared. We need to alert patients to the fact that some care is delivered by others and that they need to be briefed on the patient's concerns.
- Demonstrating a non-judgemental attitude towards the patient's expressed distress, confusion, anxiety or related emotions. The patient is in the midst of change and making sense of a problem requires time and support. If we empathise with the patient's concerns, we establish respect for their situation.
- Using open questions, that is questions that cannot simply be answered yes or no. So it is better to invite the patient to describe their pain, for example, rather than to ask them, *are you suffering any pain?*

- Showing attentiveness to what the patient says. That means sustaining eye contact and reserving a little time to hear the patient's account. We can confirm what we have heard and understood if we periodically summarise what we think the patient's concerns or expressed needs are. *So you're currently uncertain about surgery, because you've had an infection and your chest feels tight?*

We might, in some instances, formulate checklists or risk scales, areas of assessed patient experience that we ask about and that helps us to appreciate what requires our attention. The notion of risk scales is familiar in pressure sore risk (e.g., Satekova et al., 2017), but they are used extensively too in assessing risk of depression and suicide (Ceccarini et al., 2014) and these rely on questions that explore current patient perceptions. Sox and Stewart (2015) describe how structured questioning can extend to planning a whole package of care. Alternatively, we might combine some specific questions on the signs, symptoms and events that they have encountered, with some rather more open questions about their experience of the same. So what have you noticed about this illness? How have you felt about what is happening? Howell et al. (2018) describe the value of this when supporting newly diagnosed myeloma patients.

Activity 2.4   Speculating

Pause briefly to imagine that you are a patient who has been admitted to hospital under ambiguous circumstances. You've experienced symptoms to which you were unaccustomed. Your daily life has been interrupted by events that raise questions about your health. What do you think (from the patient perspective) are the relative merits and limitations of the opening conversation approaches outlined above, using a checklist of standard questions, following a questions algorithm and the invitation to report your experiences and feelings as you see them?

An outline answer is provided at the end of the chapter.

Early conversations with patients have multiple purposes.

- We have both to gather information that serves a clinical purpose (e.g., assessment of risk, diagnosis of problem),
- and which serves a patient and personal purpose (that which assures them, which helps to build trust) (Price, 2017a).

The balance of approaches used within the opening conversations will indicate to the patient how we see them. As a patient, are we also seen as a person? As a patient, are we primarily a conundrum to be understood? Are we quickly judged as regards what sort of patient we might prove; cooperative, uncooperative, insightful or relatively ignorant? Combining specific clinical questions associated with signs, symptoms, events with more general open questions associated with patient experience certainly appeals to patients. This approach quickly registers an interest in the person. It enables the nurse to check what they may already suspect about common patient concerns. But, for nurses, it does also raise a potential fear. If I emphasise patient perceptions too much, if I focus strongly on experiences and needs, can I adequately address all subsequent patient expectations? Being professional involves having an explicit regard for and interest in the person, while also being methodical and well organised with regard to addressing the risks that they might face.

It is unrealistic in early encounters to weight conversations entirely one way. If we focus entirely on information gathering for **clinical need**, then care is likely to seem cold. If we focus entirely upon establishing a regard for the patient as a person, then we might set in train expectations of service that are unrealistic. A patient who is incrementally invited to take greater responsibility for their care, who is asked to partner the nurse in an active way, may be less likely to progress in the desired way if the early emphasis is solely on patient-perceived needs. A different mind set may be required, focussing on the mutual understanding of changed circumstances, that which analyses the clinical problem and which marshals shared resources to address that.

Activity 2.5 Speculating

Now imagine that you are a patient who is being admitted to hospital on a pre-planned basis. How does that change your expectations of what would seem good opening conversations with healthcare professionals? How might this shift the balance of conversations between that enquired about by the nurse and that enquired about by the patient? The nurse reassures but the patient might assure as well. What might a patient wish to tell the nurse about?

An outline answer is provided at the end of the chapter.

Asking patients open questions about their experiences to date has very important benefits. It expresses a due concern for the patient and an interest in their perceptions. Understanding another's experience, their take on events, impresses as immediately human. But there is a difference between simply asking questions and actively listening to patients when they report what has happened and how they have felt (Browning and Waite, 2010). To actively listen to a patient, to hear what they tell us, requires that we have to ask questions about the significance of what is said. So, for example, a patient shares a startling interpretation of their illness – *I think my illness was cast on me, I was cursed.* Culturally, such an explanation of illness might be normal in some societies, but it is unusual in a Western one. If the patient explains this to us, teaching them about disease processes and self-care may be more difficult later. We might have to gently counter their explanations of the causation of illness. Many other patient narratives, however, are much more subtle than this. They may refer to levels of patient confidence, their hopes and aspirations, it may refer to their perceived stage of recuperation, and it is important that we note these, as it may later determine the extent to which they are able to partner the nurse in care.

Listening to, and hearing, the narrative of the patient about what has happened, what they think is happening and how they feel, is critical if the nurse is to build a rapport with the patient. But the speed at which that narrative can be known and understood varies considerably (Price, 2017a). Very ill patients, those less able to take stock of their circumstances, are less well placed to share clear narratives. We have to continue inviting the patient to recount their perceptions throughout the course of their care.

Understanding the patient narrative is very much about getting to know and to understand the patient. The appreciation of how they think about events, illness, injury, what is involved in being a patient, to begin recovering or adjusting, is important for the next stage of care work. Patients have very individual notions of the **patient role** and how they should adjust their relationships with others when ill (Segal, 2017). They may expect to behave quite passively. They may prefer to treat the illness problems in a quite rational, even a dispassionate, manner (*I am intelligent enough to manage this, so let's get on with things*). Some patients find the illness experience quite bewildering and may be catapulted into a crisis where they express wild ideas about what has befallen them. Certainly patients who suffer from major psychoses may struggle with this problem, a disordered way of reasoning about their circumstances, strange experiences and beliefs, especially as regards their ability to control their lives.

So the nurse has to take stock of the patient's ability to reason their changed circumstances. In many cases we are able to confirm that the patient is relatively well equipped to make new sense of circumstance. For example, a patient who has a pre-planned admission to hospital, or a regular visit to the clinic where we work, may have extensive knowledge of their illness and experience in managing the challenges that it throws up. Patients who undergo regular and lengthy treatment programmes may become expert about it, especially in the useful coping strategies to overcome resultant difficulties (Carmichael and Bridge, 2017).

Taking stock of the patient's readiness to share discussions of care is essential, but sometimes neglected. The pace of requirements associated with managing risk advance ahead of the patient's readiness to take partial charge of the same. The nurse becomes trapped by the need to convey information to the patient that they have some doubts about the patient's capacity to process. In these circumstances the care planning work, that which builds confidence in the patient, enabling them to feel in charge of events, lags behind risk management demands. While we must gain informed consent to proceed from the patient wherever possible, it is not always true that the decision making can be as ruminative or as widely debated as we might like.

I can now summarise the important work of hearing the patient narrative (Table 2.1).

Reason	Notes
To establish the patient history, what risks the patient faces.	We listen to the patient story to understand the sequence of events, to identify patterns within the illness and the risks that they pose.
To understand patient perceptions, fears, needs, hopes and aspirations.	Illness is an experience and the patient is likely to respond to us on the basis of this experience. The better we understand patient perceptions the more sensitively we can respond.
To express interest in the person and develop a rapport.	The way in which we respond to narratives signal much about our concern for the individual, our respect for the person.
To establish what the patient anticipates as regards their perceived role.	The patient comes to care with different notions of what the patient role is. The better we can understand this, the more effective and supportive our guidance might seem.
To ascertain the emotional and the reasoning state of the patient.	Much of care involves shared thinking and learning, but we need to ascertain the emotional and the reasoning state of the patient through what they share. A patient in shock, confused or in pain, for example, is much less able to partner the nurse in care.

Table 2.1   Reasons to hear the patient narrative

Sharing risks and identifying desirable ways forward

The next relationship work that the nurse does with the patient is to explain risks, the clinical imperatives to consider particular options, and to balance this with an exploration of patient preferences. Classically, the person-centred care literature has tended to treat the latter in terms of major treatment protocols, to elect choices, for instance, over whether to pursue surgery or to continue more conservatively with support or pharmaceutical measures (Adams and Grieder, 2013).

However, not all care planning negotiations relate to the larger treatment options. They may relate, for instance, to rather discrete measures such as, for example, administering their own injections. Understanding how to give yourself an insulin injection involves an assessment of drug calculations, an appreciation of why injections are needed at set times and how this balances food intake and exercise levels. What is important, however, is that the nurse honestly relates the requirements of successful risk management alongside respecting the patient's wishes relating to how they proceed. In the example of insulin injections, it is a necessity that they learn to manage their own insulin treatment regimen.

Whatever is argued within the healthcare literature about person-centred care, the patient's right to help shape care, and issues relating to the management of risk and effective use of evidence, at the patient's bedside they all come together. Care is not an either/or matter; nurses have to help patients shape their care but not to the undue detriment of their safety. A patient might wish to persist in his or her lifestyle habits, those that manifestly undermine their health. In such circumstances, the nurse cannot stand back from alerting the patient to the possible costs of their decisions.

Activity 2.6   Reflecting

Think of a patient that you have cared for, where clinical risk management and patient preference (expressed need) appeared to be in conflict with one another. How important was it to explain the risk in full; the possible consequence of actions taken or neglected? How important was it to learn about the patient's specific fears in searching for a solution that would meet both risk management and person-centred care objectives?

An outline answer is provided at the end of the chapter.

Much of the shared care decision making centres, though, on what is good/safe/advantageous to do and what the patient feels that they can relate to, cope with, succeed in (e.g., Bewtra et al., 2014). A balance has to be struck between the two. Insisting that patients completely change without due consideration of their ability to adapt may reassure the nurse that she has *told the patient what is required*, but it doesn't necessarily assure success. In practice, outcomes achieved, courses of action agreed, are a compromise, that which minimises risk and which maximises the patient's confidence that they can achieve and sustain the planned change.

Activity 2.7   Critical thinking

How do you currently think about risk in health? Is it in absolute terms? Risk is to be avoided at all costs! Do you instead see risk as a calculation?

First, there is the perceived likelihood of something coming to pass (e.g., the wound breaking down and gangrene setting in), a calculation we might call the 'likelihood of penalty'. If we don't act, or act in the wrong way, this might result.

Second, there is the perceived significance of that event occurring (e.g., what the event entails, perhaps losing a leg and becoming wheelchair-bound). We can call that calculation 'the significance of consequences'. Risk can be described in terms both of the likelihood of costs and their significance if

(Continued)

(Continued)

they occur. The way in which nurses think about risk and help patients think about risk is part of what counts as person-centred care. It helps the patient to realise their share of responsibilities in care decision making.

As this answer is based on your own observation, there is no outline answer at the end of the chapter.

Agreeing roles and what counts as progress

The analysis of risks and felt needs, the preferences that the patient has regarding how to proceed, describes shared care work. It describes what the parties think needs to be done and quite probably their sequence as well. But two other questions remain: who will do the work involved and, second, how will we know that it is working as expected? Polit and Feiring (2016) remind us that the nurse's work in rehabilitation can remain problematic and that this is precisely because of differing expectations of role. Determining what we do, and what we ask the patient to do, is not always straight-forward.

Imagine a scenario in a care home, where elderly residents are getting ready for a planned social event. All might agree that the patients are dressed as comfortably as possible. Morale is sustained where patients feel well dressed for something shared. The challenge is that this agenda also includes sustaining the maximum level of independence. The more the resident manages to do things for themselves, the greater the support for their self-esteem. So now nurses must decide how much to guide dressing and how much to do things for residents. Is the nurse the guide and support or is she the task completer? In practice, nurses negotiate compromises. The nurse may put the patient's socks and shoes on for them, appreciating how difficult that is for infirm patients. Other dressing steps (putting on a shirt for example) count as desirable self-care skills. While it might seem less person-centred to do work for patients, less dignifying, it might not only be a logistical necessity given staff resources, but it might also be something that reassures the patient as well. Ageing is not only a psychological process, it is also a physiological process as well. The capacity to affect all areas of self-care is gradually encroached upon.

The clarity of roles that nurses adopt is important in person-centred care. Where a nurse seems to adopt different roles and to change these from shift to shift, the patient might have difficulty knowing what to expect. Care can then seem ambiguous, inconsistent. One nurse seems to expect this of the working relationship and another nurse expects something entirely different. It is important, then, to identify the roles that we try to play with patients, to relate this to the perceived level of care partnering that they seem to be ready for, and then to act in consistent ways.

Activity 2.8   Reflecting

What roles have you played with patients? Jot them down now. How important did it seem to explain to the patient what you were trying to contribute? How important did it seem to be consistent in your approach?

An outline answer is provided at the end of the chapter.

Table 2.2 outlines some of the roles that nurses adopt with patients. Importantly, the roles that nurses can adopt are influenced by the patients' ability to partner care, the length of the available care relationship and the nurse's skills. Not every role is available to all nurses, nor does every nurse feel confident in every skill, so continuing professional development may have to focus on priority skill deficits within a team. For example, in a setting where patient self-care is important to manage chronic illnesses, the role of educator becomes especially important.

Role	Notes
Problem analyst	Early in the care relationship patients may need assistance to describe a problem that they face. Naming it, describing its features, deciding its extent is usually a prerequisite to solving it. For example, a patient might need help to characterise their incontinence and the associated fears that they have.
Counsellor/ advisor	Counselling involves many different things and it can be practised at different levels, dependent on the education, skills and facilities available. Here, however, I refer to very modest possible courses of facilitated reasoning. Most nurses are engaged in this work, helping patients to weigh the merits and the limits or costs of different courses of action. For example, the nurse might help the patient deliberate on the merits or otherwise of using antidepressant medication for an additional three months.
Educator	Nurses teach patients a variety of skills, but they are often more than trainers, working to help the patient build confidence in their own ability to enquire and go on learning beyond the care environment. To help others learn is to help others think in new ways and to determine what seems to work well. For example, the nurse teaches a service user (learning disabilities) how to plan and cook a meal, taking precautions associated with heat sources and reviewing what is valuable about different foods.
Confidant	Patients vary widely as regards their support network, the people available to reassure them that they are worthy of respect, praise and love. In many instances the nurse reminds the patient of their dignified endeavours, dealing with adversity and change. They listen to the doubts of the patient and signal respect for what is being attempted. For example, the nurse helps an 8-year-old to take stock of what is involved in sustaining friendships when chemotherapy has induced alopecia. The child fears that friendships will surely be lost.

(Continued)

Table 2.2   (Continued)

Role	Notes
Motivator	One of the things that patients often record as especially valuable is the encouragement that nurses provide. Assuring the patient that he or she is doing well is especially valuable when the nurse refers to what is commonly managed in these circumstances, at this stage of recovery or rehabilitation. A 'well done' that is referenced against what is usual or normal 'by now' can be especially valuable. For example, an elderly man is helped to appraise his progress post stroke by the nurse explaining what has been achieved over time when improvements have often tailed off for other patients.

Table 2.2   Possible nurse roles in a person-centred care relationship

The roles outlined in Table 2.2 are especially psychological, those that give focus to shared care work with the patient. They don't supplant the 'looking after' work of the nurse. For periods of time, nurses will need to perform care activity for the patient that they would routinely manage themselves. Person-centred care still delivers hands-on physical caring, but there comes a point within care when 'doing for' the patient is not as valuable or needful as 'doing with' the patient.

Patient **motivation** is critical to the success of person-centred care. If some of the care work is to be owned by the patient as much as the nurse, then it is necessary for them to learn indicators of progress. The nurse knows what other patients achieve, and they also know what is reported in the literature, but patients may be ignorant of this. So, as part of the negotiation of care, patients need assistance to ascertain what reasonably counts as progress (Sanderson, 2014).

Nurses quite often think of progress markers in terms of what patients can do. We often find it easier to remark on patients' progress in mobilising for example. In some rehabilitation settings we might even record progress using video recordings so that the patient can see how much more that they can do. But person-centred care is both physical and psychological. A patient who has suffered burns, for instance, makes progress not only in terms of their wound improving in appearance and function but also with regard to how they talk about themselves as well (Dunpath et al., 2015). A patient might start with feelings of disgust at their changed appearance and then gradually adopt a more practical way of talking about a new, a more resilient, sense of self that is based on a sense of humour and stoicism.

Activity 2.9   Evaluating practice

Think back now to the roles that you played with patients, those made in response to Activity 2.8. How easy was it to set down markers of progress in each of those? For example, if you acted as a motivator, what could you highlight to the patient, which suggested that they had achieved a more positive outlook on their future?

An outline answer is provided at the end of the chapter.

Learning lessons, adjusting plans for the future

The final stage of work brings the nurse back to where they started, anticipating the circumstances and the needs of future patients. Much of that work is best done collectively with others, through case discussions, discussion of audit results, participation in local research projects and so forth. But there is personal reflective work to do as well and some of this is usefully the focus for continuing professional development and registration update work. Imagine a situation where you have noted some recurring challenges met by patients preparing for surgery. Perhaps the focus is upon anxiety and the different ways in which patients conceive of lost control, trusting to anaesthesia and to the skill of the surgeon. Following through on those cases in order to write up insights from the experience of offering an individual support to patients would form a coherent focus for critically evaluated practice. Price (2017b) has highlighted the value of writing up such case studies for publication within the professional press.

Learning lessons can be thought about in different ways. Nurses have frequently been encouraged to think of this work in terms of judged performance. We articulate what we got wrong and what we did well. While such honest evaluation is important and a necessary critical examination of practice, it is not the only focus for learning lessons and adjusting plans. One of the things that clinical experience often teaches about patients is not just how diverse they may be but how patients change during the care relationship. A patient who was entirely passive at the start of a relationship becomes incrementally more confident. They become increasingly more assertive (Ludman et al., 2013). At issue here is how we learned to read the patient's changing response to the support that we provide. How did we read that which worried and that which reassured them?

The important point here is that patients teach nurses about the interpersonal aspects of care. If you are willing to listen, to observe patient reactions, to think again about how a dialogue developed (what they said, what you said, how that affected our shared work), you can start to appreciate how nuanced care sometimes has to be. It is not, then, that you succeeded or failed perhaps, but rather that you discover how a discourse (our shared understanding of need, of direction and progress) changed over time. If patients tell stories of their experience, then you may come to share stories, joint ones created by patient and nurse together. *We tried this and that didn't work. We thought about involving some other people at this point, but the patient wasn't confident right then.*

Activity 2.10 Reflecting

Have you ever been privileged to take stock of care work with a patient in the above discourse terms? Jot down what seemed to facilitate that. Was the

(Continued)

(Continued)

patient especially reflective; comfortable with reviewing joint efforts made to solve problems? Did the patient seem expert on their own illness, so that you felt free to learn things from them? Understanding what makes for good evaluative circumstances might prompt you to ask patients to anticipate such stock taking as care progresses.

As this answer is based on your own observation, there is no outline answer at the end of the chapter.

While the adjusted care identified by teams of healthcare professionals might represent a major change (for example, the replacement of some equipment, a different way of teaching patients about a therapy) that connected to your individual practice, it is often much more discrete. So perhaps you listen and respond in a different way. One of the ways in which I learned to listen was to think of my responses as a two-step affair. The first was usually to register that I had heard what was said and that it seemed significant to me. I might say, *so you are really worried about making matters worse, doing the physiotherapy. You're unsure what your leg can stand after that operation.* Here I am registering a concern for the patient's fears, but I am also specifying what I understand. The patient has doubts about how the operation has affected their leg. The second response, though, was usually to imagine what might help the patient. I would speculate, thinking aloud with the patient about what might alleviate their concern. *So, maybe we talk to a patient I know. He isn't an athlete, he wouldn't describe himself as confident, but he has completed the physiotherapy work and tested out his leg. How might that seem?* What is interesting about the recurring second responses that I often made was that they didn't promise something that I would necessarily give or do. They were increasingly phrased in terms of what we might try.

Chapter summary

In this chapter we have explored what person-centred care might consist of if we insisted upon a very practical, a local and a collaborative attitude to it.

A pragmatic approach to person-centred care comprises:

- different sorts of work – person-centred care develops through stages, that which is planned in advance of the patient's admission, that which centres on their **narrative** and that which moves on to assessment of risks and the agreement of roles;

- it focuses on a process, an explorative one which involves responsibilities for each party – person-centred care, in this sense does not abandon standards, protocol or policy requirements, those strongly linked to risk management, but it does encourage patients to play their part, sharing their experience of illness or injury, problem or need, and their perceptions as to what might represent support and collaborative care in response to that;
- the nurse focusses on both clinical and felt need – the nurse must alert patients to risks and requirements associated with an illness and/or treatment as well as diligently attend to the patient's hopes and aspirations.

What is vital within this expression of person-centred care is preparatory work. That which the team of practitioners does in advance to understand the recurring concerns and needs of patients represents an investment for the future. It enables nurses (and others) to convey their expertise and experience quickly to patients, and their compassionate concern for what worries patients. It enables the nurse to focus enquiries with patients in a much more strategic way. That learned from evidence is used to pursue care enquiries with patients that may pay greater dividends as the care relationship develops. The patient may conclude, *the nurse knows about this situation so well. They find the time and interest to understand how I encounter it too.*

Activities: Brief outline answers

Activity 2.1   Critical thinking (p27)

Much of the appeal of seeing person-centred care in terms of work focusses on the fact that we know this concept well already. We go to work. We collaborate with others to achieve strategic ends. At work, people bring different skills to bear and they have different roles to fulfil. Work indicates something in progress. Work varies day to day and sometimes it is more successful than at other times. Arguably person-centred care is much the same. It relies on collaboration and the identification of what colleagues wish to achieve. While ideals, standards and protocols all exist, it is through renewing engagement each day that work becomes real, something that we have the potential to feel good about.

Activity 2.3   Reflecting (p29)

One of the best clinical placements I completed as a student nurse was on an oncology ward where patients received a variety of chemotherapy treatments. It would have been very easy to have seen the patients purely in terms of the side effects of drugs used to treat them. But my mentor immediately asked me to tell her three other psychological concerns that patients might have that were not focussed on their medication. I offered a couple of suggestions but what impressed me was that her concerns were more about coming into hospital, being away from home and changing roles because of feeling sick. Her placement briefing to me started from the perspective of the patient journey.

Activity 2.4   Speculating (p31)

From my perspective I would hope to note two things. First, that a group of the questions seemed well ordered and linked to references made in my notes or care plan. I'd want to feel that important answers were clearly recorded and the questions were methodical. These would tell me that the nurse understands my problems. But I would hope too to be asked questions about 'my take' on what was happening. This would reassure me that the nurse was interested in my experiences. Interestingly, it seems much harder for nurses to record points about such patient perceptions. They are harder to summarise in notes, perhaps because nurses fear that they don't represent the patient fairly. What do you think?

Activity 2.5   Speculating (p32)

I wonder if you agree with me that a higher percentage of standard questions and explanations might seem acceptable in the pre-planned admission circumstance? Why is that? Perhaps as a patient the very fact that the care ahead for staff is routine, well-practised and familiar might seem reassuring. I might feel that the staff are confident that nothing untoward is likely to happen. I will have some queries that I want answering, for sure, but I might be quite content to listen to quite a lot of standard explanation of care ahead. It's worth remembering that questions from healthcare staff can signal things to patients beyond respect and reassurance. Lots of questions might, for example, indicate uncertainty on the part of staff; that they're unsure what is happening to me as a patient.

Activity 2.6   Reflecting (p35)

I remember caring for a patient who regularly used marijuana to manage his joint pain. The man suffered from arthritis and had periodic bouts of joint inflammation. However, his conception of marijuana as 'medicinal' clashed with the physician's fears that the patient's reasoning ability was becoming progressively eroded. The patient spoke in a slurred way and protested that his 'weed and booze' were not hindering his ability to self-care. As a result of this a contest slowly evolved about whether we cared about the patient's pain and whether alternative medications recommended were in fact an attack on his use of marijuana. It became critical to explore with the patient the incremental side effects of his preferred drug. But that had to be done with clear respect for his own coping strategies.

Activity 2.8   Reflecting (p37)

I used to counsel patients on problems they faced after major trauma such as burns. My expertise was in altered body image care. One of the things that I did was to take the patient shopping for clothes. This had a threefold purpose. First, it enabled them to practise their encounters with the public when they felt disfigured. Second, it enabled me to help them review what clothing styles seemed more functional (for instance, getting arms into sleeves could be difficult if keloid tissue limited shoulder movement). Third, it enabled me to discuss clothing colour and profile with them. The design of their clothes either accentuated their disfigurement or helped disguise it. It could draw attention to a deficit or distract gaze away from it. So I explained that my help on these visits was as social encounter support, practical try-out clothes advisor and appearance psychologist.

Activity 2.9   Evaluating practice (p38)

Referring back to my answer to Activity 2.8 above, progress markers were of two kinds. There were things that the patient stated about how they felt, how confident or otherwise they were with regard to managing encounters with others, and things that I observed. Sometimes the two were not in kilter. For example, a patient might state greater confidence in coping, perhaps out of gratitude for my help. But their actual ability to manage a social encounter was much less. They avoided contact or withdrew very quickly indeed. So I would start with encounters that required less interaction. We would watch the news with other patients in the TV room, sitting at the back. It was a short encounter and one just a little less face to face.

Further reading

The three texts recommended here are all chosen to help you contextualise what is involved in delivering practical person-centred care. Much of person-centred care is expressed in psychological terms, so reading texts such as these will equip you to approach patients in a more sensitive and empathetic fashion.

Aaslestad, P (2009) *The Patient as Text: The Role of the Narrator in Psychiatric Notes 1890–1990.* Oxford: Radcliffe Publishing.

It might surprise you that I am recommending a book by a Norwegian literature professor (the book is published in English). But pause to consider just how important narrative and narrating are in mental healthcare practice. This is a book that connects person-centred care and narrative intimately together, and it is (I think) relevant to colleagues beyond the mental healthcare field.

Fishman, S (2012) *Listening to Pain: A Clinician's Guide to Improving Pain Management Through Better Communication.* Oxford: Oxford University Press.

Pain represents an excellent illustration of the need for healthcare professionals to work closely with the narrative provided by patients. Whatever we think pain associated with an illness or injury might be like, patients quickly remind us that pain is experienced and expressed individually. Dipping into this textbook you should be reminded of the requirement for pragmatic person-centred care.

Ofri, D (2017) *What Patients Say, What Doctors Hear.* Boston: Beacon Press.

There is a risk that we only hear from patients what we expect to hear from them. We start with a 'mental set' as regards what illnesses and treatments signify to patients. This useful book challenges the assumptions that we might bring to care encounters.

Useful websites

www.nationalvoices.org.uk/person-centred_care_in_2017_-_national_voices…

National Voices represents a group of different UK charities who advance the interests of patients. In 2017 they published research on the extent to which healthcare service users felt that services were meeting their needs in a person-centred way. This link brings you to that report.

www.bmj.com/content/350/bmj.h181

This link brings you to Eaton et al.'s (2015) article entitled 'Delivering person-centred care in long term conditions' published in the *British Medical Journal.* The article outlines some of the challenges associated with delivering person-centred care, which emphasises the sorts of work related here in Chapter 2.

www.nice.org.uk/guidance/sg1/chapter/patient-centred-care

This link takes you to the National Institute for Health and Care Excellence (NICE) guidance on person-centred care, published in July 2014. Significantly, NICE characterises care requirements as recurring or periodic. Do the NICE guidelines support the case made for preparatory thinking about commonly recurring patient needs introduced in this chapter?

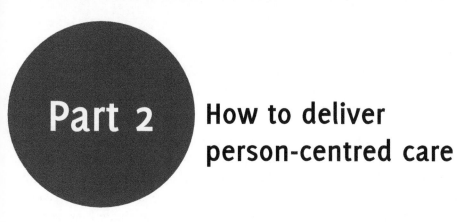

Part 2

How to deliver person-centred care

Part 2 of this textbook comprises seven case-study-based chapters, each of which focusses on the application of the different elements of person-centred care work outlined in Chapter 2.

In Chapter 3, attention focusses upon helping a patient to make sense of their circumstances and the case study centres on a woman who is being investigated for signs and symptoms of multiple sclerosis. This is aided by the work of hearing the patient narrative, the better to understand their perception of current circumstances.

In Chapter 4, attention shifts to helping patients cope with change and anxiety. In this chapter the patient has moved beyond the first sense-making activity and they now confront the anxieties that attend a diagnosis of bowel cancer. The work elements addressed in this chapter include hearing the patient narrative, sharing risks and identifying a way forward.

In Chapter 5 you are guided on helping patients to learn about treatment, care and recovery. The chapter explores the business of learning and the nurse as a person-focussed teacher. Once again, I will detail some of the anticipatory patient concerns and needs of such patients, but I will also focus on the work of agreeing roles.

Chapter 6 is entitled 'Helping patients to rehabilitate'. To rehabilitate can seem a fearful exercise. The person-centred care work featured in this chapter centres on the managing of patient fears, agreeing roles associated with rehabilitation and learning from the patient's experiences as they complete exercise and lifestyle-adjustment programmes.

In Chapter 7, I move to the business of helping patients build and sustain self-care motivation. If the preceding two chapters have focussed a great deal on teaching and supporting patients in a person-centred way, then this chapter is about helping the patient to sustain motivation once they have left the nurse's acute care support. In this chapter I will draw on preparatory work associated with understanding depression and patient motivation and then concentrate on the work of learning lessons from our work with the patient, adjusting care so that it is better suited to their future support.

Chapter 8 is focussed on care of the dying and it features a case study of a young boy who is dying from an inoperable brain tumour. In this last case study I explore how best to help the child and his mother to cope with this. I draw together all the kinds of work that you read about in Chapter 2 of this book.

I conclude Part 2 of the book in Chapter 9, reviewing what it takes to orchestrate person-centred nursing care and looking forward to the future. There is no case study associated with this chapter as I instead consider some of the opportunities and challenges ahead. A number of factors suggest that the care relationship is already changing, but person-centred care is not vouchsafed unless we anticipate how best to use our insights and skills.

Chapter 3 Helping patients to make sense of their circumstances

> ## Chapter aims
>
> After reading this chapter, you will be able to:
>
> - understand the practical working of person-centred care at the start of a support relationship and when the patient is still making sense of their circumstances;
> - understand the ways in which the nurse draws on the narrative of the patient and evidence of patient need gleaned to date.

Introduction

Chapter 2 of this book detailed the different sorts of work that nurses must engage in if their care is to be pragmatically person-centred. I begin the case-studies illustration of that with a patient who is at the very beginning of illness, with the collection of signs and symptoms that signal that something is wrong. In this chapter you are assisted to understand the sometimes quite subtle work of the nurse as he or she helps the patient make sense of what is happening. In these circumstances it is important that the nurse anticipates the nature of patient concerns and needs. To that end, the case study nurse (Omara) makes good use of evidence. But it is important, too, that she listens attentively to the ways in which the patient tells her story. What the patient focusses on and how she explains her circumstances and priorities offer vital clues on what the patient would find most supportive.

In the United Kingdom in 2018, some 100,000 people have been diagnosed with multiple sclerosis, with an incidence three times higher in women than men (MS Society, 2018). The incidence of multiple sclerosis worldwide has been estimated to be 2.5 million cases (Ghafari et al., 2015). Of those diagnosed with multiple sclerosis in Britain, 85 per cent are likely to suffer from the remission–relapse form of the disease while 15 per cent suffer from the progressive and more aggressive form from outset (NICE, 2016).

Multiple sclerosis is a disease of adult years and frequently first presents in people who are in the midst of their working and reproductive years (Sillence et al., 2016). However, the progression of the disease, the extent of relapse, the frequency of relapses and the degree of residual infirmity varies widely (Isaksson and Ahlström, 2008). It is therefore the quintessential case study for patients who are trying to make sense of their circumstances. Not only can the first and sometimes mild signs and symptoms of the disease prove ambiguous and difficult to diagnose, but the repeated bouts of illness can be readily ascribed to other causes. By the time that the patient receives a magnetic resonance imaging (MRI) screening check, diagnostic of multiple sclerosis in 90 per cent of cases (MS Society, 2018), a range of signs and symptoms may have been experienced.

Multiple sclerosis is a degenerative neurological condition that affects the insulating myelin sheaths of nerves within the nervous system and it produces a wide variety of signs and symptoms. These include fatigue, pain, unsteadiness of gait, difficulties with urinary bladder or bowel control, problems associated with sight, altered sensations such as neuraesthesia or paraesthesia and psychological problems such as anxiety and depression (Murray, 2017). The pattern of relapse is unpredictable and the length of relapse and residual difficulties left as a result of nerve scarring varies widely.

Activity 3.1   Speculating

Imagination is an important aspect of person-centred care, envisaging how patients perceive their circumstances. So now imagine that you have suffered a series of illness bouts that have come and then gone over the last 18 months. Importantly, these affected different parts of your body and they lasted for only a short period of time before resolving without medical treatment.

Make some brief notes in response to the following questions.

1. How do you habitually make sense of signs or symptoms that concern you but then seem to disappear?
2. Who might you share your experiences with and why? Is it automatic that you consult a doctor?
3. How is the experience of illness and your response affected by the fact that these events arise during your productive working-life years?

An outline answer is given at the end of this chapter.

Human beings are regularly affected by variations in their health that raise their level of concern, but which, if they subsequently subside, might be explained in ways that serve to reassure us. For example, blurring of vision might be ascribed to excessive computer screen work. Viruses are frequently used to explain bouts of unexplained illness. We, for instance, say that we have a cold or flu, but we don't work out exactly what caused the problem. To say that someone is debilitated by a 'bug' is to acknowledge that they feel ill, without searching for a precise cause. However, a pattern of recurring illnesses might cause greater concern (see Figure 3.1). We may link the bouts of illness and say that we are 'run down'. But the likelihood of such connections being made are dependent upon whether they affect the same part of the body and whether the signs and symptoms are similar (Murray, 2017). Medical consultation is more likely if we recognise a pattern to the illnesses. Those linked to multiple sclerosis might not seem obviously of a pattern and someone without medical training might find it much harder to make connections between them as they relate to a body system operating in different parts of the body.

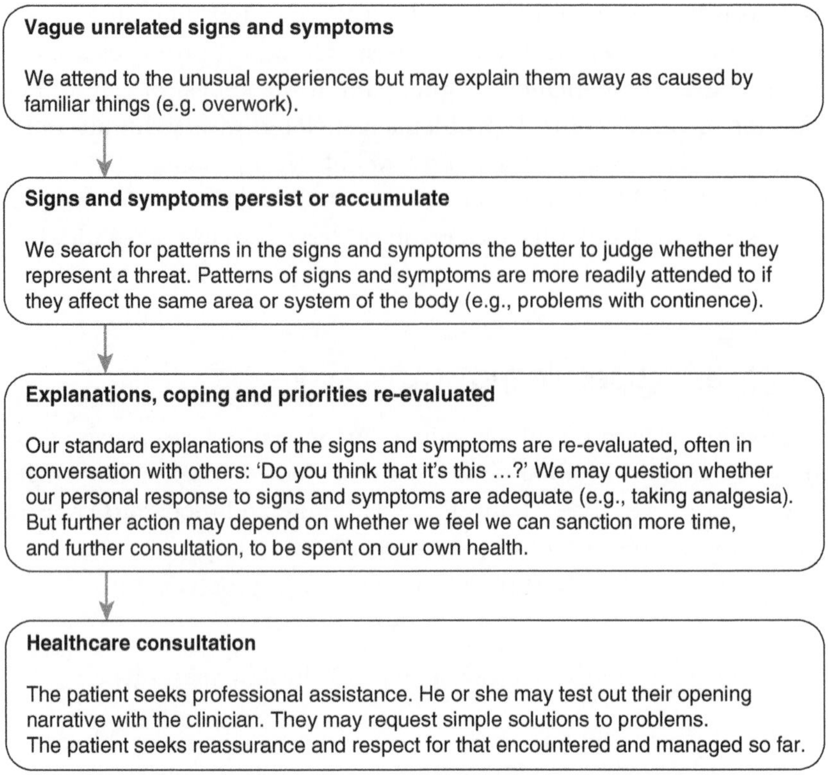

> **Vague unrelated signs and symptoms**
>
> We attend to the unusual experiences but may explain them away as caused by familiar things (e.g. overwork).

> **Signs and symptoms persist or accumulate**
>
> We search for patterns in the signs and symptoms the better to judge whether they represent a threat. Patterns of signs and symptoms are more readily attended to if they affect the same area or system of the body (e.g., problems with continence).

> **Explanations, coping and priorities re-evaluated**
>
> Our standard explanations of the signs and symptoms are re-evaluated, often in conversation with others: 'Do you think that it's this ...?' We may question whether our personal response to signs and symptoms are adequate (e.g., taking analgesia). But further action may depend on whether we feel we can sanction more time, and further consultation, to be spent on our own health.

> **Healthcare consultation**
>
> The patient seeks professional assistance. He or she may test out their opening narrative with the clinician. They may request simple solutions to problems. The patient seeks reassurance and respect for that encountered and managed so far.

Figure 3.1 Making sense of first signs and symptoms of illness

Human beings narrate their illness (Jurecic, 2012). They produce accounts of what is happening or has happened and what this means. The narratives used might come from past experience of illness or injury, or they may be constructed by a little searching on the internet. Patients may ask their associates, neighbours and friends what they think is happening to them. However, by the time that patients reach a medical consultation, they may have a host of possible explanations for their symptoms, some of which are inaccurate but nonetheless are believed to be plausible. Alternatively, they may decide that they know what is wrong and seek medical help to treat it. Patient narratives at this early stage of care are important for a number of reasons. They may:

- signal something of the distress, anger or other emotions felt by the patient;
- suggest what attitude the patient takes towards the illness;
- portray what the patient currently does or does not understand about their circumstances;
- indicate, in a preliminary way, what the patient might value as helpful.

To illustrate some of this we turn now to a patient. Megan is a 31-year-old married woman who works part-time as a teaching assistant in a school. She is married to Sean who works at a factory. The case study summarises events but, more importantly still, it offers passages of Megan's experience expressed in her own terms. Those passages are presented in italics. Attending to them, speculating on what they convey, is at the heart of person-centred care when patients try to make sense of their circumstances.

Case study: Megan

During the course of the last 14 months Megan has been concerned by three bouts of illness, none of which she has connected up as indicative of an underlying problem but all of which she has associated with feeling 'generally under the weather'. Megan is the mother of twin boys aged five and she works in the infant school that they attend. Because Megan is good at her job and has a passion for education the deputy headmistress has mentored her in preparation for a teaching course, which would enable her to take charge of a class of her own. But the mix of preparatory reading, working in class herself and raising her family with Sean has seemed unrelenting pressure for Megan. Sean tries to help but Megan describes herself as 'Mrs fix it'.

Fourteen months ago Megan suffered some unsteadiness of gait. Her legs ached and she complained of pain in the small of her back. She described it as feeling as though *one leg was shorter than the other.* A little before that time she had played netball with friends and while she couldn't remember a specific injury, she ascribed her problems to a sports injury.

It's easy to pull your back in netball, because of all the sudden twisting and turning that you do. At any rate, I thought about my aching back, the discomfort in my legs, my wobbliness and I thought, you've strained your back. I felt stupid over doing it when I have so much to do. Sean was a bit concerned and said that sometimes people pushed a disc out of place. I told him not to fuss. If the problem kept on I'd maybe see the doctor about it. I suppose, honestly, I didn't want to sound selfish, whining about a sports injury when there were really poorly people. So I rubbed in some Voltarol (an anti-inflammatory cream) *and gradually it all seemed to get better. I couldn't be doing with reporting sick when I'm busy.*

Seven months ago a further bout of illness affected Megan. She noticed that her eyesight was blurred. The problem seemed to start quite quickly, so she was alarmed at first. Sometimes the blurred vision was accompanied by headaches. Around that time Megan had embarked upon a programme of reading about child development and learning. Her mentor had recommended it as an excellent way of checking out whether a teaching career would suit her in the longer term.

I made excuses again didn't I. I assumed that my eyesight problem was to do with eye strain. I was reading a heck of a lot of material then and some of it was quite difficult. Anyway, I made excuses for myself, started to search for an optician to visit in case I needed glasses and I told Sean that he would have to work extra shifts because none of those things come cheap. Then Sean had his accident at work, slipping on the engine oil. He dislocated his shoulder. My fuzzy vision got forgotten and slowly it seemed to improve by itself. I simply read a bit less and cooked and cleaned a bit more.

It was in the last month though that Megan suffered the bout of illness that prompted her to visit her GP. Megan noticed that she had weakness in her hands. It was difficult

(Continued)

(Continued)

to grip a pen or pencil to show the children how you formed clear letters. Her arms felt painful too and there were sometimes pins and needles down her right arm.

I visited my GP and he told me to grip his fingers, just to test how strong my hands were. He put my arms through a range of movements and then he asked whether the pain was worse if the weather was cold. He started moving my head around and checking my neck. He asked me about whether I'd had an injury, did I ride a horse maybe? I laughed and said no, I couldn't afford that! It was when he asked about an injury that I told him about my unsteady legs earlier and how I'd thought that was due to a netball injury. He asked whether I had suffered a sports injury and I said not that I could remember. That was when he started asking more things about my health in the last year or so and after that he referred me to a nerve specialist. He said that they might do a scan that could help identify what was causing me all the problems. I looked at him I did, and asked why he said 'all these problems'. Well, he told me that they might be linked. I might have nerve inflammation, that was how he put it.

It is important to study the whole of Megan's case, not only what happened to her but also to assess how she tells her story. The account that she gives concerns not only the experiences of illness, but how these related to the rest of her life. That which happens physically affects how she thinks about herself and her role, as a wife/mother and as a teaching assistant. The account also refers to what happened when she visited her GP and what he told her about her worries. Notice, for instance, how often Megan's assessment of problems is referenced against her role responsibilities and what can be afforded. Notice too how the medical explanations have been understood, *nerve inflammation*. Megan has a propensity to set her own health needs aside and to hope that problems will resolve themselves. It is only when she cannot do what she is paid to do that she feels justified in asking for help.

Megan visited the neurological specialist in the local hospital and he arranged for her to undergo a magnetic resonance imaging (MRI) scan. He explained that she would need to spend a little time in a rather large and imposing machine that might feel claustrophobic. She would have to keep very still until she was told that she could move again. Completing this test would enable him to 'exclude multiple sclerosis' as a cause of her problems.

Activity 3.2   Reflecting

Jot down your own impressions of how Megan tells her story of illness and her first encounters with healthcare professionals. To what extent is she currently able to make sense of the situation? How alarmed or anxious do you think she seems? How would you characterise the process of learning about what her signs and symptoms could represent? We will return to your notes later in the chapter.

An outline answer is given at the end of this chapter.

Anticipating the concerns and needs of the patient

As was explained in Chapter 2, anticipating concerns and the needs of the patient by researching or auditing past patient experience is a valuable thing to do. While there are many questions that you could ask patients like Megan, you can begin to focus down your enquiries and your explanations if you know what patients are commonly concerned about.

Omara Cooper is a clinical nurse specialist dealing with neurological deficits at the district general hospital that Megan visited. Omara works with the neurological ward at the hospital, but also with the outpatient department through which Megan came for her MRI scan. While there are lots of other specialists who meet women like Megan, technical, medical and therapist colleagues, it is the clinical nurse specialist who works most closely with patient experience. She helps patients to tell their stories so that the personal understanding of illness as well as the health deficits met can be revealed. Omara became sensitised to person-centred care through her work with patients suffering from sickle cell anaemia in the Caribbean. It taught her that illness was personally interpreted. Forever afterwards it made her curious about how illness was constructed in the minds of patients. That which seemed important to patients often suggested a good place to develop a rapport.

When she met Megan at her MRI appointment Omara elicited the account you read about in the case study. But she also brought to the support of Megan a great deal of preliminary work that she and colleagues had done before. If Megan related experiences and perceived problems in her patient history, then the preliminary work done on multiple sclerosis and patient uncertainty by healthcare colleagues would inform what Omara could use to explain possible events that might unfold in the future. Making sense of illness involves interpreting past events and trying to anticipate future ones.

While Omara knew that there was a significant chance that Megan did suffer from multiple sclerosis (given her history), it was by no means certain that this was the only possible diagnosis. Medicine proceeds stepwise, excluding other diagnoses, using the patient history and various tests in order to describe the challenge that the patient faces (Kornelsen et al., 2015). The problem for patients is that the planning and sequencing of tests follows a diagnostic rationale that isn't necessarily linked to patient experience (see Figure 3.2). Women like Megan encounter signs and symptoms, changes to what they can do, and they receive competing informal explanations of what 'was wrong with you'. The diagnostic procedure focusses on body function more than personal experience. Patients experience illness in terms of levels of acuity (how bad it seems right now) and in terms of perceived levels of uncertainty. That contrast of foci is especially true of a neurological condition such as multiple sclerosis, which offers an accumulation of worries that, over time, cannot so easily be ignored. In Omara's experience, patients emotionally judged their opening responses to signs and symptoms. There was a risk that Megan might feel guilty for not having sought help sooner. She might worry that, by delaying investigation and diagnosis, she had somehow allowed the condition to get worse.

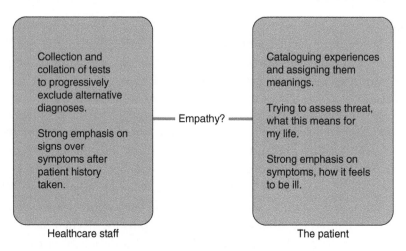

Healthcare staff

The patient

Figure 3.2 Parallel processes (diagnostic steps versus patient needs)

Activity 3.3   Reflecting

Discuss with colleagues whether you, as a patient, have sometimes retrospectively judged your early handling of a health problem that was 'brewing'? How judgemental were you of yourself? Have you ever anticipated that negative self-evaluation in patients that you have supported, and have you sought to explore with the patient whether their self-criticism was warranted? What message do you think is given to a patient when you anticipate that which they have already judged about themselves?

An outline answer is given at the end of this chapter.

Turning to the multiple sclerosis patient experience research that Omara had read, there were a series of issues that she understood might be of concern to a patient such as Megan. The first of these started with MRI scanning, that which Megan has come to complete. Patients have a number of fears relating to the MRI scan experience and these are not necessarily associated with what the tests will confirm. They were to do with being inserted into a machine that made strange noises. Patients such as Megan wonder how something this big can look inside the body without in some way changing it. They wonder what sensations they may experience while inside the machine. One of the patients that Omara has cared for described it as an hour inside a washing machine, which sounded as though it was *processing you in some way*. The same patient associated *big machines* with cancer treatment. Particularly disturbing was the fact that the patient is left inside the machine, the attendants retiring to operate it. Brand et al. (2014) have described how patients have been educated to manage this, and how they have taken away a computer disc on which are their own scan results. The goal was to help the patient manage the experience, but having receipt of technical information is not effective unless it is explained to them. For that reason, Omara takes a different tack and describes the scan in a stepwise fashion, always with regard to what the process will *seem like. That's what's really important isn't it, envisaging what will happen and how it will probably seem. This isn't a ghost train ride!*

Activity 3.4   Critical thinking

The National Institute for Health and Care Excellence (NICE) standards (2016) for the early stage care of patients with multiple sclerosis make provision for a number of things. For example, patients should receive a face-to-face consultation with an expert physician within six weeks of diagnosis. Thereafter there should be a single point of contact person for the co-ordination of their care. Treatment of any multiple sclerosis relapses should start within 14 days of the problem being reported. What, though, do you think is missing from standards that describe the maximum time that a patient must wait, or whom they can expect to consult? What does Omara add for Megan in the way she describes the experience of having an MRI scan?

An outline answer is given at the end of this chapter.

One of the things that Omara noted from experience with past patients was how often the explanation of multiple sclerosis omitted reference to pain. Patients frequently referred to their fleeting pains as soon as she asked about how they had been feeling. While there is explanation given of how the disease process damages nerves, and the rationale for drug treatment, much less attention was given in the literature to patient discomforts. Yet in a study by Vidovic and colleagues (2014), most patients studied reported one or other form of pain that they associated with multiple sclerosis. Omara's experience also suggested that some form of pain was relatively common in the early stages of multiple sclerosis and that it was important to ask about this, recording what the patient reported. Also, asking about pain was for patients a vital indicator of whether healthcare professionals cared about them.

While Omara had to decide just what she discussed at each stage of illness with a patient, one of the recurring concerns of patients did need to be addressed from the outset. This concerned the support that they might receive. Expectations of support differ and people report differing experiences.

- Nickerson and Marrie (2013) had noted that patient and physician assessments of treatment, for example, often differed markedly, with healthcare staff assessing it a lot more positively.
- Patients with multiple sclerosis face the risk of depression and they tend to grieve each loss of physical function (Isaksson and Ahlström, 2008). Initially patients felt extremely vulnerable and they then struggled to develop a sense of control.
- Patients tend to receive much more support during the diagnostic and first treatment phase of the illness. Support tends to drop away afterwards. In response to this Dennison et al. (2013) commended Cognitive Behavioural Therapy to help patients to develop successful coping strategies.
- Solheim et al. (2017) observed that patient evaluation of opening support was often positive but evaluation of later support was much less so. Reporting on when patients deteriorated further, Davies et al. (2015) described how patients felt that they were *just left to get on with it.*

In Omara's experience patient dissatisfaction was often linked with disappointment that staff didn't imagine how the illness would seem in the longer term. The dissatisfaction with support was much less when a different mind set was established from the outset, one in which the nurse and the patient saw themselves as joint problem solvers. Teaching patients about their condition and treatment was not enough. It was important to help them to think positively about how to use information and to go on learning and consulting (Borreani et al., 2014). While the nurse had a responsibility to respond quickly to the patient, there was also a responsibility for the patient to catalogue their experiences and their own problem-solving efforts en route. This meant that patients saw themselves as less the victim and more the manager of health requirements. Oeseburg and Abma (2006) described this as seeing care in 'mutual endeavour' terms.

Because of this, Omara gently explored the possibility that the scan might reveal that Megan suffered from multiple sclerosis and she said that, if it did, then they could work together on some shared solutions over the years ahead. What Megan hadn't consulted a doctor about earlier in her illness was not the key determinant of success in the future. What determined future success was how they thought about the problem together.

Activity 3.5 Critical thinking

Decide what merit there seems to be in Omara anticipating the nature of the illness ahead and the advantage of seeing it in joint problem-solving terms. How do you think Omara's understanding of how service provision is often experienced might seem to Megan? You might debate whether Omara should discuss multiple sclerosis before a diagnosis is confirmed. Some patients might prefer to deal with one problem at a time, but others might insist that forewarned is forearmed. At issue here is whether Omara appears to be a better support if she brings experience and expertise to bear quickly. The doctor has already indicated that they are investigating whether Megan has multiple sclerosis.

An outline answer is given at the end of this chapter.

Hearing the patient's narrative

One of the risks of clinical nurse specialist work is that the expertise of the nurse relies increasingly on the nurse's understanding of diseases, investigative processes and treatments. To patients, that expertise might seem rather technical or cold. Once a treatment regime has been identified the nurse commends it firmly. There is a sudden shift towards prescription. For patients this can seem quite unyielding. Sheridan et al. (2012) have described how expertise can seem daunting. Patients dealing with chronic illness may be especially prone to feeling that their experience does not count as much as other kinds of evidence.

Omara's counterbalance to this, however, stems from research into patient experience (see above) and a growing catalogue of narratives that patients suffering from multiple sclerosis have shared. While she is duly cautious of typifying how patients experience the disease, she acknowledges, too, that some recurring accounts are at least identifiable and that these in turn may shape how a patient hopes to be supported (see Table 3.1). This ability to spot the patterns of thought is something that seems instinctive to her. You learn to spot the early signs within a narrative that suggests ways in which patients think about their circumstances and, from that, you start to determine what counts as a need. While disease risks suggest a clinical need, patient narratives about experience suggest patient needs.

Narrative descriptor	Notes
Illness as something to be accommodated within a positive life.	The illness is fitted into a lifestyle, the patient searching for ways to reach accommodations between the demands of the two. Efforts are made to limit the distractions of illness upon the patient's preferred lifestyle.
Illness as a life change.	The patient redefines their life in terms of coping with the illness. Real or anticipated problems and responses dominate life planning.

(Continued)

Table 3.1   (Continued)

Narrative descriptor	Notes
Illness as retribution.	Illness is perceived as a penalty for beliefs, actions or attitudes adopted in the past. The patient may or may not relate this to religious beliefs about sin or proscribed lifestyle. The patient embarks on a review of good living as well as coping with the illness.
Illness as a status, a focus for expertise.	The patient studies their illness extensively, the better to understand it and anticipate what happens next. It is important to the patient that their developing expertise is recognised by healthcare staff.

Table 3.1   Possible patient narratives associated with multiple sclerosis

Activity 3.6   Critical thinking

Look back to the notes that you made in response to Activity 3.2 and the narrative that is shared within the case study above (pp51–2). Omara thinks that one of Megan's needs is likely to centre on the effects that multiple sclerosis might have for her family and work responsibilities. Megan thinks of herself as a 'doer', someone who responsibly supports others. So, whatever else Megan might worry about as regards the prognosis of multiple sclerosis, a focus of concern for her will be upon sustaining her work in helping others. What above leads you to support Omara's first assessment?

As this answer is based on your own observation, there is no outline answer at the end of the chapter.

It might seem strange to think about a diagnosis such as multiple sclerosis in terms of its impact on work or family function first, because the nurse understands so much more of its damaging effects on the body. We anticipate incapacity, fear, anger, a centring on feelings of vulnerability. But Omara has picked up from Megan's narrative that she habitually puts the needs of others first. Megan starts from a different place to the textbook concerns that we might associate with multiple sclerosis (Murray, 2017). This is not to dismiss those classic personal concerns, but it is to acknowledge that they might be tackled in a different order. To use a simple analogy, the nurse must start to solve the jigsaw with the patient by using the pieces that are handed to her. What might enhance trust is that which manifestly stems out of the history that Megan has shared and the implicit priorities that are signalled there.

Why is Omara confident that this early focus on the social/work impact of the disease will seem supportive to Megan? You might have noted the following:

- that Megan seems to see herself as too busy, in fact, to attend to health worries of her own;

- that what prompts Megan to visit her GP finally is that which materially limits her ability to teach – she sees herself as a helper;
- that she doesn't dwell on more concerning explanations of difficulties in her legs – a prolapsed intervertebral disc is a significant risk to wellbeing and future function, but Megan sets the alternative explanation aside;
- that Megan is passionate about teaching and plans a career there – multiple sclerosis has the potential to disrupt that career.

An early nursing instinct is to give patients a great deal of information. The simple formula used is that uncertainty prompts anxiety and anxiety in turn is resolved by giving more information. This can seem a reassuring approach for the nurse because they then feel that they have delivered a service. They have informed the patient about matters. In practice, however, during the period while the patient is still making sense of circumstances, the art is in sharing the information that seems most useful to the patient. You ascertain where the patient starts from in their sense-making process and begin there, rather than from the gamut of information that might be relevant and the delivery of which might enable you to feel expert. So, in this instance, the amount of information that Omara shares with Megan about multiple sclerosis is based on the patient's sense-making needs.

The next extract is a small part of the dialogue that Omara shares with Megan, that which explains something that the MRI scan could reveal and that tries to link this to what Omara understands might probably be a felt need of the patient.

Megan: *So the scan could prove that I have multiple sclerosis ... is that what my doctor meant by nerve inflammation?*

Omara: *Yes, multiple sclerosis is a disease that damages nerves, by inflaming and scarring their coverings. That can be why hands feel weak, or legs feel unsteady. It can explain the pain or unsteadiness that you have noticed.*

Megan: *And that comes and goes ... like what happened to me?*

Omara: *Yes, the disease can flair up. The scan you are having can show a lot of detail about parts of the nervous system that are damaged in some way.*

Megan: *But it goes away again?*

Omara: *Quite often, yes, but it can return and the awkward thing is that we don't know exactly when or how often.*

Megan: *That's scary. That's pretty scary....*

Omara: *You were telling me about all you have to do. You're going to be a teacher I think? There are the boys to consider too? The uncertainty of when the illness flairs up would be a big worry?*

Megan: *Yes, that's right! That's right. I'd have to think hard about that ... the not knowing when it was coming back.*

Omara: *If it is multiple sclerosis, planning becomes awkward. But I think you and I can plan for eventualities. For example, there are many ways to teach, many teaching posts with varying amounts of commitment for instance. If you had multiple sclerosis it doesn't mean you can't teach and help people. The patients I know don't feel that they should let the disease make them wait for the next problem. They say, I'm going to get on with things.*

Megan: *It's about attitude.*

Omara: *Very much about attitude. I can't imagine … you allowing yourself time to feel sorry for yourself. Would you say that's true?*

Megan: *You're right! I'm way too busy.*

Omara: *So if it is multiple sclerosis we tackle it that way. Planning what you need to do. Planning how you can use our help to do what you set out to do.*

Megan: *Yes, thank you.*

Activity 3.7   Critical thinking

Look back at the short extract above and answer the following questions.

1. How does Omara use her insight into Megan's opening narrative to focus her help for Megan?
2. How much information does Omara share about multiple sclerosis at this stage and what does that focus upon?
3. Why do you think Omara emphasises attitude towards illness so much in this conversation? How might that appeal to Megan?
4. Given your responses to Activity 3.1, how do you think Omara's explanations and suggestions would seem to you?

An outline answer is given at the end of this chapter.

Person-centred insights

I will now review some of the most important insights into person-centred care available within the case study of Megan.

Sense making as a process

The first of these insights is that the sense-making narrative of patients increases incrementally and that it comprises of layers of experience, speculation, insight and concern. The patient starts with signs and symptoms and the pattern of illness encountered. While in healthcare assessments you might concentrate more on signs (they seem more objective), patients often concentrate more on symptoms. Megan reads her bouts of illness in terms of how they felt and what that seemed to be associated with (her functional ability). *My vision is 'fuzzy' so I can't now do …. My hand feels weak, so I can't help children with ….* Recognising the experiential nature of illness at this stage is likely to increase the chances that a patient feels that you understand and respect them.

Understanding patient concerns

The second insight is that your assumptions about the level of patient anxiety might not always be accurate. In this case study, Megan expresses a growing concern about her health, but she does not concentrate on her own wellbeing. Concern is not necessarily the same thing as personal anxiety. This is a significant matter because where you believe that anxiety levels are high, you might be tempted to reassure patients with more information. What is more important in the sense-making stage of illness is often the reading of how the patient thinks about their situation, and using the right information (Stone, 2014; Olaug and Robson, 2017).

Clinical needs and patient needs

It is important to distinguish at this first encounter stage between clinical needs and patient felt needs. Clinical needs are usually associated with managing risk or ensuring that the service seems effective and efficient. You need to work strategically with the patient so that they achieve as much independence as possible. Patient felt need, though, comes from the very process of change, in this instance the incremental sense making of illness, its ability to alter how we live. That has implications for the preparatory work that you do to assist patients who use your service. The research and case studies that you read or collect need to focus on patient experience as well as on disease processes. If you read research on a disease and ignore the illness then there is a greater likelihood that the ways in which you respond first to the patient seems system centred rather than patient centred.

Recognising patient perceptions

Attending carefully to the narrative of the patient, not only what they say but also how they say it, enables you to estimate how the patient perceives their circumstances. It is not an exact science and you might misinterpret patient concerns, but failing to make this assessment will probably seem worse. In our example, Omara has amassed a range of insights into patient experience and need from research and local case studies, but she still attends carefully to what Megan says about her patient history. That Megan focusses so strongly on her responsibilities to others is materially significant. Megan is likely to deal with multiple sclerosis by valuing her own coping in terms of what she still manages to do. What Omara deduces from Megan's narrative will help shape what information she offers.

Anticipating patient needs

One of the key things Omara emphasised within her opening work with Megan was that the nurse should not prematurely judge the discourse that the patient was sharing. While you should search for patterns within patient narratives, i.e., the typical ways in which needs were thought about, it is necessary to avoid stereotyping the patient. In this case study, the discourse might well prove to be *seeking assistance with that which enables me to serve others.* But this discourse could change again, especially were Megan's illness to move from a remission–relapse format to something more aggressive and constant (Davies et al., 2015).

While Omara emphasises an explorative approach towards Megan, through the analysis of the narrative Omara has a clear conviction about supportive care. Because chronic illness demands that, later, the patient self-manages much of their care, there is a greater need to conceive of care as collaborative and partnered from the outset. It is inescapable that the patient will need to become involved in some problem-solving work.

Working differently

Sometimes nurses wonder whether they have the time to personalise care, especially at the start of collaborative care work. They may fear that to deliver person-centred care is not only to make promises that the service cannot keep, but to also spend a great amount of time exploring patient perceptions of need. In practice, however, the need for greater input is sometimes overstated. Instead, the nurse attends differently to what is already offered in a patient narrative. Notice in this case study what is carefully surmised from the way in which Megan describes her circumstances. While more questions could be asked and sometimes are, there is much to glean from comparatively short narrations. Notice too how Omara discusses what the MRI scan might reveal. She doesn't share significantly more information about multiple sclerosis at this stage, because a patient has a right to know, she shares that information that seems to connect best to what she understands Megan's opening concerns to be. In sharing an attitude towards illness, that which other patients use with success, she offers the message, *we can deal with this, even if it does prove difficult.* A patient leaving this care encounter might reasonably feel that Omara has not only been interested in them, but that there is a prospect of hope as well.

Chapter summary

Helping patients to make sense of their circumstances represents an exacting test of the nurse's ability to approach patients in a person-centred way.

- It involves working with a body of well-established information regarding the possible diagnoses that the patient might receive and what the chief challenges and concerns will be. What the nurse studies in advance needs to relate to both clinical needs (e.g., those related to risk) and personal felt need (i.e., the ways in which patients typically confront and cope with an illness).

- However, the nurse must attend closely to the narrative that the patient offers about their experiences to date. These attest to the ways in which the patient has been making sense of signs and symptoms, whether they identify a pattern there, and whether that causes the patient anxiety or simply a growing concern. Learning to read the way in which a patient tells their story can help the nurse to ascertain what information they hope to receive first.

- Conditions such as multiple sclerosis represent a profound and lifelong threat to the wellbeing of a patient. But the way in which that is made sense of is likely to be quite individual.

- While, conventionally, care begins with open questions, those that allow a patient to share their perceptions and communication techniques alone do not establish rapport. The nurse has to quickly attend to that which the patient reports with greatest concern. They also have to anticipate for the patient the challenges that could arise ahead.

Activities: Brief outline answers

Activity 3.1   Speculating (p49)

1. I wonder whether, like me, you develop a number of different working explanations, personal narratives, to explain the signs and the symptoms that you encountered? Symptoms in particular can seem ambiguous, worse one day than another. We might argue that a skin rash (a sign) is either there or not there, but symptoms can seem a little more ambiguous.

2. We know that patients often try out their account of illnesses with a variety of lay people before they consult a clinician. In sociological terms, this is not because the person consulted is a medical expert but because the individual is someone who we believe to be reasonably rational. This is an important narrative because, when the patient seeks medical help, they may already feel guilty about not consulting professionals earlier.

3. You may, like me, have referred to a narrative about whether a working adult feels that they can afford to be ill. You may believe that significant illness is associated with old age. For such reasons it can be easy to set aside signs and symptoms and to 'soldier on'.

Activity 3.2   Reflecting (pp52–3)

Do you agree that she prevaricates on accepting that her illness is potentially serious? As a nurse, you may have already been taught to read clusters of signs and symptoms in order to profile a potential disorder that the patient suffers from. At first, Megan is not unduly anxious about her circumstances, although she clearly hopes that whatever affects her will not hamper her. Patients are not always immediately anxious unless their first signs or symptoms of illness are dramatic (as, for example, in a myocardial infarction with sudden chest pain). Megan is then still at the beginning of her sense-making journey. She will have to learn about the threat it poses, the limitations that it might create, but where she starts with that learning will be informed by what she worries about most.

Activity 3.3   Reflecting (p54)

Sometimes we imbue illness and our responses to the same with a moral quality. We might argue that an adult should behave this way or that. We might believe that we should not make a nuisance of ourselves at the doctors. Against that, we know that we shouldn't ignore dangerous signs, those that are best treated early. It's very likely that Megan experiences doubt about the wisdom of her past actions so supportive reassurance, i.e., the nurse showing that she anticipated such doubt and perhaps self-recrimination, signals to Megan that staff have regard for the feelings associated with illness.

Activity 3.4   Critical thinking (p55)

Omara offers a humane response to Megan's experience of ambiguous illness; she anticipates how confusing this could be. Notice how Omara describes what having an MRI scan feels like. While NICE standards (2016) are important as a description of the service that should be provided, they do not describe the interpersonal enquiry process that makes support feel individual. Omara in these circumstances is likely to ask a lot of open questions about how the symptoms or signs feel.

Activity 3.5   Critical thinking (pp56–7)

Omara understands the potential loneliness of the healthcare system. She appreciates that the early flurry of provision, around assessment, diagnosis and treatment, can raise expectations of support that are not always met later on. Megan may well feel daunted by the forthcoming monitoring and self-care work, but, while there is an experienced nurse like Omara who portrays it as a problem-solving process, there is also hope.

Whether or not you would prefer to consider possible diagnoses before one is confirmed depends on your coping approach. I prefer the 'forewarned is forearmed' approach. It enables me to feel that I have a little more thinking time, and time to manage my emotions if an unpleasant diagnosis is confirmed. But it is important to ask a patient, *how do you like to cope with uncertainties?*

Activity 3.7   Critical thinking (p60)

1. Omara quickly focusses on what worries Megan most and decides to describe something of the possible diagnosis, judging that Megan needs time to understand what adjustments she might have to make in her lifestyle.

2. Omara's description of the illness, its altered physiology, is comparatively simple isn't it. But notice the honest way she refers to the unpredictability of relapses as it is this that Megan will be strongly concerned about.

3. Omara focusses strongly on attitude because she understands the lifelong effect that a chronic and often progressive illness can have on the morale of a patient. It would be comparatively easy for Megan to see herself now as 'victim' but, given Megan's lifestyle circumstances, this is something that is unlikely to seem attractive.

4. I thought Omara's opening explanations were a good match to what Megan has described regarding her lifestyle. She has started to read Megan's character. A good way to see illness and its challenges is one that works closely with the patient's resources and here Omara is already starting to sense Megan's pragmatism. So Omara's communication is likely to seem 'can do'.

Further reading

In this case study Megan will secure a definitive diagnosis. But there are many patients, in both physical and mental healthcare contexts, who face protracted uncertainty as regards what their signs and symptoms mean. Reading about the patients' problems and needs in the following three articles will further acquaint you with what may be required.

Kornelsen, J, Atkins, C, Brownell, K et al. (2015) The meaning of patient experiences of medically unexplained physical symptoms. *Qualitative Health Research*, 26 (3): 367–76.

Olaug, L and Robson, C (2017) 'It's incredible how much I've had to fight': Negotiating medical uncertainty in clinical encounters. *International Journal of Qualitative Studies on Health and Well-being*, 12 (1): 1–13.

Stone, L (2014) Blame, shame and hopelessness: medically unexplained symptoms and the 'heartsink' experience. *Australian Family Physician*, 43 (4): 191–5.

Useful websites

By going to **www.youtube.com** and typing 'multiple sclerosis patient stories' in the search box you will secure a number of accounts of how patients have learned about their illness and coped afterwards. It is well worth studying the mix of patient responses, the better to appreciate what they have in common and the ways in which personal coping remains a very individual matter. Having dipped into the selection, I wonder how much like Megan these patients and their story-telling seemed.

A frequent YouTube contributor on multiple sclerosis narratives is a young man called Seb (*My MS Story (Life of Seb), My MS story – 2 years later*). Seb ably illustrates the very variable experience of early symptoms, the length of time that it might take to secure a diagnosis and some positive ways to respond to illness as a disease progresses. It is useful to review his video stories to appreciate how his thinking about illness changes.

Chapter 4 Helping patients cope with change and anxiety

Platform 4: Providing and evaluating care

At the point of registration, the registered nurse will be able to:

4.2   work in partnership with people to encourage shared decision making, in order to support individuals, their families and carers to manage their own care when appropriate.

Chapter aims

After reading this chapter, you will be able to:

- understand the ways in which an anxious patient might be prepared for planned surgery in a person-centred way;
- demonstrate the way in which different healthcare professionals can work together using evidence, experience and patient insight to anticipate risks and negotiate a best way forward.

Introduction

In Chapter 3 you read about Megan and a person-centred care intervention that was comparatively subtle. When the patient is still making sense of his or her circumstances, the approach of the nurse is rather more explorative. In this chapter, however, attention shifts to another early care context, that relating to patient anxiety and planned treatment.

When a patient with an intellectual disability is admitted to hospital for surgery you need to anticipate concerns, needs and requirements differently. You have to appreciate how the patient reasons and to anticipate what they might find difficult. Whatever evidence exists regarding hospital care and treatment (for bowel cancer in this case study) means little unless it is mediated by an understanding of the patient and their coping ability. If the case study of Megan represented a relatively discrete intervention, then the case study of John illustrates a more labour-intensive one. That which is done before admission is likely to pay dividends later. Thinking ahead is important in person-centred care.

Once patients have moved beyond the stage of sense making, i.e., what the signs or symptoms or test results really mean, they may enter a period of increased anxiety (Price, 2017c). Patients often find change discomfiting, so in this chapter I focus on change and anxiety, and I consider the circumstance where an older man confronts cancer of the bowel, recommended surgery (a left hemicolectomy) and the formation of a temporary stoma. Surgical treatment of this kind, for a tumour that is in situ within the bowel muscle but which shows no signs of spread beyond, offers a relatively good prognosis (American Cancer Society, 2018). It might seem obvious that the patient should simply proceed with surgery. But change and anxiety is not like that. Both are very individual, especially if the 60-year-old man deals with a moderate intellectual disability and lives within a sheltered community. John has not dealt with hospitals before, he hasn't dealt with cancer and he hasn't dealt with surgery.

Human beings have repeatedly to make sense of their environments, to manage what might otherwise seem an overwhelming amount of new information. To address this we use memory, storing past events and registering them as either threatening or reassuring. The amygdala (a part of the brain intimately involved in risk assessment) operates with the memory to determine what deserves our greatest attention (Price, 2017c). That which has seemed threatening in the past, which was associated with unpleasant sensations and difficult outcomes, is likely to receive considerably more attention than that which seemed unproblematic. Pleasant experiences we might be drawn to as a matter of habit, but unpleasant ones represent a risk, a cost and we have to think much more carefully about how we will proceed. Because human beings cannot realistically process every new event as something fresh, we tend to build and rely on template explanations of what an event means (Owen, 2014). We assign those situations where the events seem very familiar to one of those templates. It is this that allows us to focus our attention then on things that seem strange, to consider that which seems more ambiguous.

Activity 4.1   Reflecting

What, within your experience, supports the argument that we rely on template reasoning? When you have cared for patients how apparent did template reasoning seem? Did you have to enquire about how patients thought of an illness, an operation or a health change?

An outline answer is given at the end of this chapter.

One of the problems for patients facing hospital care and treatment is that they might not have a template to which to refer. For patients dealing with an intellectual disability, significant change, like admission to hospital, like surgery, like treatment for cancer, represents an especially challenging problem. This is so for a number of reasons:

- the change may occasion acute anxiety in a patient who may already be predisposed to feel anxious;
- it may mean that the patient tries to rely on past templates that are inadequate for the change before them, so that their responses to staff then seem odd, ignorant or even belligerent;

- it may threaten an overload of information and new learning demands within a short space of time;
- it might make the patient feel trapped and less able to work with others.

Patients dealing with an intellectual disability are more likely to suffer from anxiety (Nelson and Harwood, 2011; Reid et al., 2011; Hermans et al., 2013). Those, for example, dealing with a condition within the autistic spectrum are especially prone to anxiety (Keefer et al., 2016). A patient with a moderate intellectual disability, one with more reasoning ability, might imagine many more threats associated with a prospective change than one who has severe intellectual impairment (Hermans et al., 2013). There is a need to plan for these events, to enable the patient to rehearse what is going to happen, so that the strangeness of change is limited. There is a need to plan for the admission to hospital and for nurses working in intellectual disability and oncology care to work imaginatively together.

Case study: John

John is a 60-year-old single man who has, for the last ten years, lived within a sheltered community supporting people with intellectual impairment. John worked in a local hotel. In this work John was well-liked and respected, although, as he got older, his ability to organise his day became progressively less. John is of a cheerful disposition, but he is certainly fearful of anything that disrupts his regular routine.

As part of a screening programme for older men, John was checked for abnormal cells or blood within the stool. The investigators called him to clinic with his regular support worker Alice. Further investigations were carried out that Alice explained in terms of whether his gut was working well. John knew about guts as, when working at the hotel, he had cleaned fish and rabbits in the kitchen. The doctor gently told him that he had a cancer of his gut, but that the tests revealed that it was limited to the muscle and that if a portion of his gut was cut out, then the disease could probably be removed. The doctor explained that for a while he would have a 'bag on his belly' to collect the poo, but that, later, another operation would mean that he could use the toilet again in the normal way. It was possible to 'mend his gut' if he had an operation very soon.

While the doctor simplified his language, Alice observed that he attempted to share too much information with John in one go. Learning that he had cancer, that he needed surgery and that this would lead to him having a bag on his belly, were three major changes that John wasn't ready for. He needed to process the information a little at a time, so Alice arranged to rehearse with him these matters as three stories, becoming ill, even though I don't feel poorly, needing to go to hospital and have an operation, and, then, being different in the way that I go to the toilet. The days after John was advised of his serious illness were difficult for John and for Alice. He became tearful

(Continued)

(Continued)

and withdrawn and Alice noticed that he didn't want to eat with the others. John said that there was *something wrong inside me because of my eating and that it was best to eat alone in case something went wrong.* So Alice arranged to share some meals with John, and it was during these that she encouraged him to describe what he feared.

Here are three short excerpts of narrative that John shared during their conversations. The first concerned the causation of cancer. John knew people sometimes did get cancer but he didn't have an accurate idea about why it happened.

When you eat the wrong things then that can make you ill. You mustn't put things in your mouth that are bad for you. I don't know what I ate that's bad, I don't know what I did wrong, but I don't want to do it again and I don't want the others to see me as bad because of it.

John's conception of the aetiology (the origin or cause) of cancer was limited. He knew that fibre was good for you (*your greens*), and that you could get ill if you didn't eat those. He knew that people sometimes suffered from tummy problems through eating germs. But he also seemed to identify a moral origin for the cancer, as though he was being punished for not eating properly. Alice was aware that some of John's reasoning templates centred quite strongly upon his mother, whom he missed. Much of his early life had been directed to pleasing her and it seemed possible that she monitored his diet closely.

The second excerpt of narrative was associated with hospitals. Going to hospital could be necessary for quite small things: *people get their gall bladder out, Dorothy did.* But he was aware too that sometimes hospitals kept you there a long time, something that worried him intensely.

I suppose they decide how long they going to keep you once they have you there. They decide for you and they keep you till they ready to let you go home. I don't know how strict they are, whether you can ask to go home, but I expect they might say no. They won't let you go until they are ready.

Alice noted the heavy emphasis on rules as John talked about hospital. He assumed that they were rule-governed places and that there was little scope to please the patient. Rules John liked, but those were rules that reassured. Rules that kept you away from friends might be bad rules.

John's third narrative concerned the *bag on your belly*. He had no clear conception of what this was or how it related to protecting the bowel while recovery from surgery proceeded. The cutting of bad bits out of you didn't seem entirely strange as he cleaned fish and you cut things out that weren't good to eat, but he didn't understand how he would pass poo onto his tummy and that he would need to change the bags attached so as to remain clean.

I don't know much about bags and your belly. What do you carry around at any road? What you put in that bag and why you have to carry it? I reckon that they cut a hole in you and they take out the bad bit. Then they sew you up. You don't need a bag, they take the bad bit away.

John has completed his pre-assessment clinic, during which the doctors assessed his physical health, his readiness to undergo anaesthesia and to spend up to 12 days in hospital. In two weeks' time John will come in for surgery, and he must be ready to give his best informed consent to surgery and to anticipate what his hospital stay will entail. Alice meets Kieran who is going to be John's link nurse when he comes onto the surgical oncology ward. They are going to plan how to help John deal with this change.

Activity 4.2   Critical thinking

Identify what you think John's reasoning templates are in the above case study. How adequate do they seem to help him? Alice and Kieran agree that they need to improve John's expectations of what will happen and to minimise the complexity and threat of the change that hospital is for him as much as possible. Jot down why you think understanding a reasoning template is so important if care is to seem personal and respectful.

An outline answer is given at the end of this chapter.

Anticipating the needs and concerns of the patient

In planning John's pre-hospital support, Alice and Kieran have access to several bodies of research evidence. The research evidence that they highlight in their discussions relates to bowel cancer (stage 2) and surgical treatment, to anxiety among people with intellectual disabilities and to helping such patients to manage a hospital admission. As neither practitioner has the complete review of research evidence available their consultation is very important. It is necessary to know that all the relevant information has been considered.

The threat of cancer

Bowel cancer represents an open-ended threat to a patient (McKenzie et al., 2011). While a patient might achieve remission following treatment, an absolute cure is not necessarily assured. Instead, clinicians refer to five- or ten-year survival rates. In John's case it would be possible that his operation could be the first of several changes that Alice has to help him through.

The research evidence suggests that hemicolectomy is reasonably successful for patients with a tumour in situ within the bowel wall (American Cancer Society, 2018).

Providing the tumour has not spread to lymph nodes there are real prospects that the patient will secure a good prognosis (McKenzie et al., 2011). Surgery in this context seems like an imperative for John. While every patient has a right to withhold consent, the wisdom of doing so in this instance is dubious. While surgery leads to a stoma and involves overcoming anxieties relating to hospital admission, the alternative prospect of disease advancement persuades Alice and Kieran to recommend the operation to John.

The risks of surgery

It will be necessary to explain that there are risks associated with surgery and anaesthetic (e.g., Ikard et al., 2013; Ramanathan et al., 2015), that it may take a while for his bowel to repair and for his stoma to be reversed, but that, on balance, these risks are much less than those of doing nothing. John already knows of a patient (Dorothy) who had her gall bladder removed, so he understands that parts of the body can be safely removed and patients can return to a comfortable life. Therefore Alice thinks that this might be a good way to convey the risks and benefits. John has enough 'gut' left to do the job required, something that he might be anxious about.

Intellectual disability

Kieran has offered the bulk of information about the success rates for the operation, but it is Alice who shares information about people with intellectual disabilities and anxieties. She explains that there are risks where patients have had bad experiences and colleagues have been less successful in debriefing the experiences with a service user. Here is a summary of the research that Alice shares with Kieran.

- People with intellectual disabilities are prone to higher levels of anxiety, but their foci of concern still varies quite widely (Nelson and Harwood, 2011). Alice highlights to Kieran how John is worried about the possible length of his hospital stay and the strictness of rules that will apply there.
- People with intellectual disabilities have a much higher incidence of anxiety disorder (Reid et al., 2011). John certainly does have significant anxieties but the residential community team have assessed John and they believe that he can be assisted to deal with the hospital experience. The issue of anxiety disorder is important because a patient already suffering from that might become extremely distressed and aggressive in circumstances where they felt out of control. While this hospital episode could be managed well, Alice emphasised the need to prevent John progressing towards an anxiety disorder in the future.
- Anxiety levels can rapidly escalate for patients with an intellectual impairment. If events were unanticipated and unexplained then the anxiety levels would increase (Hermans et al., 2014). John might dwell on worrying thoughts (often unrealistic ones), experience sudden panics and these might occur when there was less to distract him. So staff caring for John at night should be especially aware of the risk.

While John's intellectual problems were quite complex, they did include features of what Kieran understood about autism spectrum disorders (Richards, 2017). John was sometimes hypersensitive to sensory stimuli, for example strange noises worried him. Monitors or drip regulator alarms could create problems. John had relatively rigid ways of reasoning. He was quite focussed on what his mother used to commend, he wished to please someone that he trusted, and in this instance that meant Grace. Grace was a local volunteer who worked with the residential community and who Alice thought possibly reminded John of his mother. It might therefore be a good idea to see whether Grace could play a role as a companion for John during his hospital stay.

Finally, Alice expressed a concern that all the staff, not just the nurses of the surgical unit, needed to respect the importance of talking with John about how he felt. This could seem a superficial concern to some doctors, something that wasn't their prime function (Adams et al., 2012). However, if members of the surgical team repeatedly failed to acknowledge John's thoughts and feelings, that would quite probably accelerate any feelings of anxiety. Kieran made a careful note of that.

Working with John's perceptions

Alice checked with Kieran about whether the hospital used a patient passport system (Northway et al., 2017). Kieran had anticipated that question and had brought along a simple one-page passport that they used (see Figure 4.1). This included three boxes that he suggested that they fill in with John before he came to hospital. The first box recorded things that John felt staff must understand about his needs and concerns. The second box related to what would help John as regards the style of communication used. For example, he might like explanations to be illustrated, either drawn or explained using an analogy. The third box related to what interested John about his hospital stay and what might enable him to feel curious about his care. Like other patients with an intellectual disability, Kieran wondered whether there were things that John might be fascinated by, eager to understand, as these could provide a greater sense of personal control. The one-page passport was attached at the front of a patient's notes, but Kieran explained that he had also arranged that a summary was produced in reduced A5 size that John could carry and show to any staff so that he didn't have to repeat his concerns. Alice was encouraged by that as passport systems are only as good as the use made of them. That which remained filed was not that which assisted the patient (Drozd and Clinch, 2016).

Helping patients with a hospital stay

Alice explained that there was growing research about the combining of storytelling (ways in which patients anticipate events that will happen) with the use of a pre-operative visit to the hospital and the use of photographs (Blair et al., 2017).

Corve Dale Hospital Passport

The following information has been supplied by the bearer of this passport and should be used in all treatment and care support measures used with them. Please take a moment to read the information before explaining any measures with the patient.

Patient's Name: *John Beddows*　　　　　　　**Patient's ward:** *Onibury*
Ward extension number: *3714/3715*

My needs

I am having planned surgery on my bowel, but this sometimes seems complicated, so if you have investigations or treatments to explain I may need simple explanation and more time to understand what you say. The hospital seems big and strange, so it's possible I could get lost. It will help me if you guide me to where I need to go. Night time in a strange place makes me anxious, so remind me where I am.

Communication

I prefer to be called John. I can hear people fine, you don't need to shout, but please talk slowly and clearly. It will help me if you avoid any big medical words. Sometimes it helps if you explain something using a drawing. Thank you.

My stay

I like flowers and the gardens around the hospital. They make me feel calm. Feelings and complicated discussions I can't keep up with. My friend Grace is a special helper who comes with me around the hospital.

Figure 4.1　John's completed hospital passport

Patients were assisted if they were rehearsed in the sequence of events, hospital admission, pre-operative care, recovery, return to a ward, as this helped them to feel a sense of control. Simple clear guides on going to hospital such as that by Hollins et al. (2015) were very useful, but Alice felt that there was value in John preparing his own scrapbook about the forthcoming visit.

Some Spanish researchers (Gomez-Urquiza et al., 2016) have studied the benefit of using photographs to help patients with intellectual disabilities to manage their anxieties. In that study, patients chose pictures of nature and of their family to prompt distracting and reassuring thoughts, and that was combined with the use of favourite music. The approach seemed to improve patient confidence and to aid recovery, when compared with simple reassurances offered by staff. Ginicola et al. (2015) had also observed the benefits of using photographs to support counselling work done with patients. Photographs could be used to help patients to focus on relevant issues and prompted a clearer articulation of their thoughts.

Kieran wondered how the different elements of preparatory care might fit together. It was routine to facilitate a pre-operative visit to the hospital for patients with special needs. That was augmented by staff members such as Alice talking over the sequence of planned events so that these were clear in the patient's mind. But what if the photographs weren't taken from elsewhere? What if the staff were willing to have John take their photographs on his pre-admission visit, so that these could be printed off and added to his scrapbook? Might that not help too, enabling John to recognise quickly those people caring for him? Was it better to use photographs to distract and reassure the patient, or to brief and familiarise the patient with people he would meet?

Activity 4.3   Reflecting

Looking back over the preceding sections of this chapter, what do you now conclude about different healthcare professionals talking about a patient's prospective care? For example, how important is it to speculate together? Next, how important is it to join up possible elements of care, those which you might invite John to consider. In this instance, that includes:

- a pre-hospital visit;
- a hospital passport;
- offer of a companion (Grace) to reassure John during the course of his stay;
- rehearsing stories of events to come;
- using a scrapbook, with photographs/images that John adds himself;
- offering music that he could bring pre-recorded to hospital, that he could play on headphones when he was feeling uncertain.

An outline answer is given at the end of this chapter.

Sharing risks and identifying desirable ways forward

While Alice and Kieran speculated about what might assist John, it was vitally important to consult with him on what might support him best. As Kieran's meeting with Alice was at the community residence they also arranged to visit John, both to discuss plans and to once again check what John understood about the planned surgery. One of the problems that attend information-giving to patients was that it was not always completely understood. Patients (in Kieran's experience) sometimes had an evolving idea of to what they were consenting.

While patients have varying capacity to understand complex concepts such as cancer and alternative treatments, the Mental Capacity Act 2005 (Brown et al., 2015) makes it clear that every effort must be made to aid patients to make decisions in their own terms. Capacity might vary from day to day (e.g., as in dementia), so it was necessary to establish that the consent being given was live and as accurate as possible. So Kieran asked John to tell him why he thought the operation was being recommended. Here is an excerpt of John's response.

Well I have a cancer inside my guts and if they don't take it away it will get worse. They say that it could block me up or else grow somewhere else inside. But if they cut it out, I got a better chance of getting better. It ain't going to stop me eating. I gotta eat the right things, but it ain't gonna stop me eating in the future.

Kieran asked John whether he thought it might be an uncomfortable operation.

They going to put me to sleep, so I don't feel it! Then, afterwards I can have tablets, they said that. They said that they would get me up soon enough, I didn't have to stay in bed all the time. I could have tablets if I got sore.

What about the bag you will wear after the operation, what do you think that will be like? Kieran wondered.

I'm going to have a bag and it must not be trapped when I do up my trousers. But I can wear it under my shirt so people don't see, John answered.

Kieran wasn't sure how much John understood about that. He knew the sort of drawings that were used to show where on the body the bag was attached. But in his experience the illustrations weren't that satisfactory. They were always seen from the front and with nothing inside them. So, checking Alice's expression, he wondered whether John might like to try a bag out. John agreed and so he unbuttoned his shirt and Kieran showed him the semi-opaque stoma bag that would be used. It had a hole in it through which the poo entered. Kieran showed how with his fingers.

Shall we make it the right weight, like it would be if you had some poo inside and needed to change the bag? Kieran wondered. John agreed and Kieran pushed a chocolate bar, in two pieces, inside the bag. They laughed, but Kieran explained it was about the right weight. John could feel how it felt against his skin. Alice watched as the filled bag was attached. She looked at it from the side. *That's why we fit the bag so your trouser waist band doesn't go across it,* Kieran said to John.

Kieran then explained how the patient passport might be a good way for John to quickly tell hospital staff what he needed, what he liked and what he was interested in. He showed John the simple format of the passport, just three boxes into which they would add information. Kieran and Alice agreed that explaining this system was a good way to open up discussions with John about some of the other support innovations that they had been talking about. Under the heading 'My needs' John certainly agreed that a visit to the hospital would help, as he worried about where he was going. He wanted to know where things would happen as well as to understand the sequence in which they would happen.

Activity 4.4   Critical thinking

Trying out something (safely, privately) is an important part of individualising care for an anxious patient. But how is Kieran using his experience here to help John? What is really wrong with a simple line diagram that shows where a stoma bag is fitted?

An outline answer is given at the end of this chapter.

Alice said, *I was wondering whether you might like Grace and myself to be your friends in hospital? We could arrange for Grace to come on the hospital visit with you, so she saw where everything was. We could then arrange for her to come with you on the day you are admitted to hospital and to spend an hour or so with you before the operation. We could arrange for her to be by your bed when you wake up.*

John's face brightened at the prospect of a friend being there during the difficult days. Alice assured him that either she or Grace would then visit daily, and talk for a good while, so that John would be able to share any worries. The support wouldn't just be for the two days. Kieran had agreed that a special friend could be granted an extended visiting time. Once again, John expressed relief that he would also have that support.

Maybe if we visit in the evening, that way we could help you get rid of worries before you went to sleep?, Alice suggested. John nodded.

Next Alice moved to the idea of using some photographs to help with the hospital visit and to help remember what was going to happen day to day after the operation. She had already ventured the idea of the scrapbook, using it to write the sequence of events that would happen as Kieran had briefed her. But text in a scrapbook alone was difficult for John as his reading ability was fairly limited. Pictures would be better. What about using pictures that he had taken himself?

John was a little more uncertain when Alice ventured decisions for him to make. This was a recurring challenge for John, one that she well understood from the past. Confront John with multiple options and the weighing of alternative actions became progressively more difficult. John felt more comfortable when decisions were branched, between two or at most three choices. Then further choices could be gradually built upon that.

Alice: *I was thinking that you could take some pictures of the hospital, the ward and the theatre when we go for the visit John? (two choices, yes or no).*

John: *We could. You got a camera then?*

Alice: *We can use my mobile phone, that takes pictures.*

John: *Right oh, yes, it does.*

Alice: *What would you like some pictures of?* (many options, but this seemed important for a sense of control and to help Kieran prepare the hospital passport).

John: *Well my bed, where I am going to sleep. Maybe the doctor?*

Kieran: *We know which doctor will be on duty for your operation John, we are going to meet him when you visit the hospital. We could take a picture together because I will be on duty too*

John: *Yes. I'd like pictures of the outside of the hospital too. I'd like pictures of the flowers if you have those.*

Alice: *Do some pictures just seem more comforting John?* (again two choices, yes or no).

John: *I like flowers. I liked putting out the flowers in the hotel reception. You take flowers for people in hospital.*

It wasn't the policy to have flowers brought to the bedside in hospital, but Kieran immediately recognised the importance of John's need. Flowers meant comfort.

Kieran: *What about if your book had pictures that helped tell your story about the operation and getting better, and we had some pictures too of all your favourite flowers. You could show them to Grace when she visits?*

John beamed. *Yes, flowers to show Grace.*

Activity 4.5   Evaluating

How well do you think Alice and Kieran are linking up a supporting friend to photographs and a preliminary visit to hospital? What is artful about the mixing of support resources?

An outline answer is given at the end of this chapter.

John liked the idea of having some music and a set of headphones to listen to it during his time in hospital. While the clinical purpose of this was to reduce the risk of panic and distress, John chose to describe its value in terms of dealing with boredom. It was nicer to listen to music. John said that he would like to take along some piano music. His mother had played the piano.

After their meeting with John, Kieran felt able to complete the hospital passport. He was quickly identifying John's needs, how he liked to be communicated with and what interested him. Whether Kieran could persuade the hospital groundsman to meet John when he was recovering, the better to see the flower beds at the front of the hospital, he wasn't sure, but he would try.

John's most pressing needs centred on a mental map of the day and how it would unfold. They could arrange for Grace to come with John on the admission day and to accompany him as far as the anaesthetic room, but, in between all the other days that Alice and Grace visited, there was a need to help John anticipate ward routine. A sense of orderliness was important to John and, while these details seemed incidental even mundane to Kieran, they were noted down as very important to John. A ward day was punctuated by meals, medical staff visits, dressing or wound checks, by the visit of the physiotherapist to help John with his chest and to start mobilising well. Kieran couldn't pretend that the ward wouldn't seem busy, sometimes noisy, so it was important to explain to John about what the staff would be doing. But there would be quieter periods too and they could adjust the lighting in the evening to help him to get ready for sleep.

Activity 4.6   Reflecting

Pause now to take stock of the level of resources needed to help John to prepare for his hospital stay. This is rather more resource-intensive than the support of Megan in Chapter 3 isn't it? But are the resources all supplied by the hospital? Is support only provided by healthcare staff? In what ways might resource use now limit the need for some resources to be deployed when John has been admitted?

An outline answer is given at the end of this chapter.

Person-centred care insights

Attending to a patient's anxiety is an excellent way to demonstrate person-centred care. But let's pause to consider exactly why that is.

Understanding patient anxiety

The first point to make is that anxiety is very individual. In some patients' cases, such as John's, the manner of reasoning is much more rigid. The scope to accommodate significant changes in events and strange information is considerably less than usual.

So, to address anxiety properly, you need to find out what causes anxiety for a patient and how that might be exacerbated by the treatment and care that are part and parcel of a hospital experience. An experienced practitioner such as Alice can explain to staff what signals that a patient such as John is becoming distressed by his surroundings. As she told Kieran, John tends to ask more and more questions when he becomes anxious. Each question must be well answered or it triggers a supplement question and that might be more exacting. There is arguably nothing more reassuring for a patient than to feel that staff have recognised the risk of anxiety and that they then respond in ways that seem to fit so well with how the patient handles change.

Certainly, the prevention of anxiety for a patient such as John requires significant planning. The effort work of professionals is shifted forward. Such work is a good investment if you consider the possibilities that could result if John's anxiety was not managed well. John might panic and become difficult to care for. More damaging still, John's memories of the hospital stay could become so negative that any future treatment needed would be much harder to deliver. In prospect there is a reversal operation for John's stoma, so that care done well now has the prospect of making the next hospital visit much easier.

Working creatively

When you pause to reconsider the consultative ideals of person-centred care, if espoused philosophically John's preference to avoid anxiety, to have a pre-set and largely predictable hospital experience poses something of a counter ideal. There are some patients who wish to confront a minimum number of decisions, who prefer to feel that others are considerately in charge. A patient such as John is perhaps not the model patient that nurse philosophers routinely envisage, i.e., one inquisitive about care options, determined to ensure that they are not only consulted on care but that it is co-directed. So Alice and Kieran must search for a middle line, ensuring that John is confronted with choices and information that register properly as informed consent, but which do not unduly pose threats to him beyond his perceived capacity to cope with change.

Significantly, in this instance, person-centred care is delivered both by healthcare professionals and volunteers. Because John's reasoning template is so closely related to memories of his mother, a voluntary worker on this occasion has a big role to play. Grace has the potential to reassure simply through her presence. The fact that she is not 'medical' and has come with him from an environment that he trusts into one that seems strange, is arguably enough to significantly reduce his anxiety. What healthcare staff have to do is to imagine the valuable role that Grace plays for a patient like John and to facilitate that role with a flexible visiting arrangement. One of the concerns expressed by staff about person-centred care is that it requires staff to do much more than they are resourced to provide. In this example, however, it may involve not revamping a service but sharing work differently.

Using others' experience

What this case study illustrates is that a great deal of the personalisation of care can rely on a knowledgeable care worker or family member that knows the patient very well indeed. In the time available to make an assessment of the patient and to build a rapport, planning how to proceed, it is important to make full use of knowledgeable others. Nurses arguably cannot always get to know patients fast enough, at least if the patient has problems with reasoning or communicating.

Nurses working in acute physical care environments may be perplexed about how best to care for patients who come to them, not only with a physical illness or injury, but also with an intellectual disability. You will become accustomed to caring for patients through specialisms and fields of practice. But a case study such as John's should reassure you that some principles might usefully apply to a wide range of patients coming from such unfamiliar backgrounds. These principles include the following.

- Work with the local care professional wherever possible.
- Establish what makes the patient most comfortable. A hospital passport helps the nurse to do that, signalling quickly what the patient wants others to understand and how they like to communicate.
- Think differently about what comforts. Historically pre-operative anxiety was often treated with a pre-operative sedative. But anxiety is equally effectively addressed by other means that seem more familiar to the patient. In this instance, this comprises of photographs of flowers and the music that the patient enjoys. A patient listening to music on headphones, thumbing through a storyline scrapbook that they have brought with them, may achieve a much better psychological state pre-operatively and better recovery afterwards.

Accessing and understanding the patient's narrative

Hearing the patient's narrative, making sense of their perceptions in circumstances such as John's, however, is much more challenging. Alice is accustomed to understanding how John reasons and she knows a considerable amount about his history. The excerpts of narrative shared in this case study illustrate that interpretation of what John says could be harder. A patient such as John has his own accustomed way of speaking. He not only uses dialect and unusual terms but he rehearses thoughts in a way that are closely referenced to his beliefs and assumptions. It might not be quite so easy to read such a patient's concerns, for instance about hospital rules and being allowed to leave hospital, unless the nurse already understands the role of rules inside John's world. It is for this reason that care, especially that associated with assessing risk and making plans, needs to be collaborative with an experienced practitioner from the patient's background or with a wise relative.

Activity 4.7   Reflecting

Pause now to evaluate your thoughts about John's case study. If your learning/work is associated with the care of physically ill patients, how anxious would you feel relating to a patient such as him? What reassurance do you draw from the wisdom of someone like Alice? If you are learning to care for patients with an intellectual disability, what does a physical care situation such as cancer and bowel surgery teach you about what you need to explain to a professional colleague about patient needs? What reassures you about the expertise of a nurse like Kieran?

As this answer is based on your own observation, there is no outline answer at the end of the chapter.

Chapter summary

In this chapter we have explored what change can mean for a patient and I have highlighted the vital role of person-centred care in assisting the patient through that change. Where a patient starts with an intellectual disability, change may be particularly daunting. The capacity to reason through change is not equally distributed through the patient population. But there are a number of points that we can make.

- Helping patients with change starts with an understanding of where they start from and to where they are progressing. Without an understanding of the patient's life context, their normal living, you are poorly placed to individualise care.
- Much associated with the support of patients through change relies upon teamwork. It is often the case that different professionals have different insights into patient need.
- There are different ways to support a patient during change and, while some of these may be resource-intensive, others can be resource-light. The engagement of a support friend in this case study is an example of that.
- Thinking outside the box and using some inspirational research can liberate care when patients are working through change. Therefore, reviewing evidence and having an advanced understanding of patient needs might prove vital to delivering exactly the right service.

Activities: Brief outline answers

Activity 4.1   Reflecting (p68)

One example of template reasoning relates to aches and pains and the use of over-the-counter analgesia. We may formulate some habitual ideas about a volume or frequency of pain that 'has to be accepted' and that which mandates medication. Sometimes the template reasoning relates to notions of what is normal, for example associated with ageing. Our template reasoning might also be influenced by attitudes towards medication and an over-reliance on pills.

Activity 4.2   Critical thinking (p71)

John's reasoning templates are poorly developed. As regards cancer he appears to believe that you either catch cancer or you at least ingest it through the wrong foods eaten. John has no conception of cell life, deterioration or the genetic base for some types of cancer. The template appears complicated by concerns that morally bad people might be more at risk of cancer. If you don't follow the rules then you might develop cancer. His understanding of hospital is equally limited. It is a place of rules, control and direction, one where control is surrendered to others. You might not be able to leave hospital quickly if you don't comply with the rules. John's template relating to colostomy and the use of a stoma bag seems to be based on simple mechanics. If you chop something out then you can join the ends together. He does not understand the concept of a bowel being rested. The templates are currently unequal to his care needs and it's likely that he could become quite distressed in hospital unless he is helped to work through what will happen to him.

Activity 4.3   Reflecting (p75)

For patients such as John staff liaison is vital. It's very doubtful that the surgical oncology team could get to know John well enough without the assistance of a support worker such as Alice. While there are a number of resources that could be used to support John, not everyone is necessarily suited to his individual needs. This is clear as regards the possible use of photographs; will they be used to divert his attention to more comfortable things, or will they be used to help anticipate the surgical journey ahead? Because John has limited ability to make sense of abrupt change, it is important that the support elements are coordinated.

Activity 4.4   Critical thinking (p77)

Kieran understands from experience that patients understand things best when they have had a chance to feel as well as see what an ostomy bag is like. It is a matter of feeling how the bag attaches to the skin and how the weight of its contents feels. Then there are the practical matters of emptying the bag and keeping the skin clean. Diagrams of ostomy bags are sanitised. Patients need to see and feel how large the bag is and what that then entails as regards wearing clothes over it. The problem with a line diagram of a stoma bag in situ is that it might not be in the place where John's will be fitted and it doesn't adequately represent the experience of wearing and managing a stoma bag.

Activity 4.5   Evaluating (p78)

Alice and Kieran are customising John's care, working with what Alice already believes will reassure John and interest him in the hospital as a place of something more than surgery. Here John is receiving different sorts of support. He will have a friend that he can talk to. He will have a scrapbook to remind him what happens next, something that is very important as he fears becoming trapped in hospital. The fact that he can use that scrapbook to talk about more pleasant things (flowers) is beneficial when a hospital rule (no bedside flowers) could have seemed threatening to him. His passport will help him to head off awkward questions that he might struggle to answer.

It's significant that Alice leads John carefully through a series of choices. This might not seem as expansive as some patients might hope for but it helps to limit the anxiety that John might otherwise feel.

Activity 4.6   Reflecting (p79)

This package of planned care is indeed rather more resource-intensive as it takes up a significant amount of Alice's and Kieran's time. But it makes excellent use of a volunteer (Grace) who John trusts and it has a realistic chance of making John's hospital stay a successful one. Given that his diagnosis of bowel cancer could lead to further hospital admissions, it seems vital that John is helped to secure a positive experience on this occasion. Some of what John does now and what he receives now by way of explanation of the ward routine may be excellent preparation for any subsequent admission to hospital.

Further reading

The notion of patients journeying, periodically, with the help of healthcare professionals has become more prominent in the literature, especially in the light of chronic illness and with a focus on person-centred care. All three of the following texts will add to your appreciation of patient experience of change and ways in which services might be arranged the better to support patients on their journeys.

Macauley, C, Powell, P and Fertleman, C (eds) (2016) *Learning from Paediatric Patient Journeys: What Children and Their Families Can Tell Us.* Baton Rouge, FL: CRC Press.

Much of the child's journey as a patient is mediated by the explanations of parents or guardians, so this is a useful source on liaising care to best effect.

Wallis, I (2014) *The Reluctant Patient: A Journey of Trust.* Arlesford: Circle Books.

In Chapter 2 (useful websites) I encouraged you to explore patient narratives of multiple sclerosis. Wallis's account continues that patient insight approach. We need to understand how patients perceive care.

Worth, J (ed) (2012) *Perfecting Patient Journeys: Improving Patient Safety, Quality and Satisfaction While Building Problem-Solving Skills.* Cambridge: Lean Enterprise Institute.

This is very much a 'how to' guide, working with patient perceptions and experiences.

Useful websites

www.theguardian.com/society/2013/sep/15/anxiety-epidemic-gripping-britain

Cooke, R (2013) Living with anxiety: Britain's silent epidemic. *The Guardian*, 15 September. Rachel Cooke's article offers some personal testimony on the experience of anxiety and how that individual links anxiety to the wider environment. It's then worth asking, how well does this match my perceptions of anxiety? Would I be more or less sympathetic to a patient who saw things that way?

Anxiety conditions

www.anxietyuk.org.uk/get-help/anxiety-information

Anxiety UK is a charity supporting people who suffer from a range of anxiety conditions and their families. This is a good site to read for a summary of the conditions and to better understand what an anxiety attack feels like. Anxiety is the lens through which change might be perceived and it is also possibly a constraint on the ways in which a patient might partner the nurse in care.

Chapter 5 Helping patients learn about treatment, care and recovery

NMC Standards of Proficiency for Registered Nurses

This chapter will address the following platforms and proficiencies:

Platform 1: Being an accountable professional

At the point of registration, the registered nurse will be able to:

1.8 demonstrate the knowledge, skills and ability to think critically when applying evidence and drawing on experience to make evidence informed decisions in all situations.

1.9 understand the need to base all decisions regarding care and interventions on people's needs and preferences, recognising and addressing any personal and external factors that may unduly influence your decisions.

Platform 2: Promoting health and preventing ill health

At the point of registration, the registered nurse will be able to:

2.10 provide information in accessible ways to help people understand and make decisions about their health, life choices, illness and care.

Platform 3: Assessing needs and planning care

At the point of registration, the registered nurse will be able to:

3.4 understand and apply a person-centred approach to nursing care, demonstrating shared assessment, planning, decision making and goal setting when working with people, their families, communities and populations of all ages.

Platform 4: Providing and evaluating care

At the point of registration, the registered nurse will be able to:

4.2 work in partnership with people to encourage shared decision-making, in order to support individuals, their families and carers to manage their own care when appropriate.

Chapter aims

....

After reading this chapter, you will be able to:

- understand how the teaching of patients about their illness and treatment might be arranged in a person-centred way;
- understand how the different conceptions of teaching relate to person-centred care.

Introduction

To varying degrees all patients become learners, something that helps shape the collaborative risk management, role clarification and progress assessment work that you read about in Chapter 2. If patients are faced with a chronic illness then learning is required. This raises important questions for person-centred care as we need to debate what is involved in the role of the learner and to consider carefully what is required of a teacher or learning facilitator.

While you may have quite clear ideas about the teaching relationship in other settings, such as college, the teaching–learning relationship in healthcare is different (Price, 2015). For one thing, the learner may find themselves in the learning role very reluctantly indeed and quite suddenly. For another, the nurse, unlike the college teacher, does not have the same powers to assess and judge the performance of the learner. The nurse's 'student' is also a consumer, and the teaching on offer represents a part of service that the patient judges. While the teaching agenda may relate to the known challenges of a disease or treatment regimen (clinical need), the patient's perceived learning needs may more frequently be linked to what the patient has felt or worried about (felt need) (Laursen et al., 2017a).

Here the nurse faces competing imperatives (see Chapter 1). On the one hand, the nurse is required to attend individually to the patient's perceived needs. On the other hand, teaching patients to self-care in the future is often vital if additional healthcare problems and costs are not to arise. Patients suffering from diabetes mellitus have to manage in excess of 90 per cent of their own care over a lifetime (Laursen et al., 2017a). Failure to take charge of an illness or disability could significantly increase the demands on resource-limited healthcare services. So, while the nurse hopes to individualise teaching, there is also an imperative that teaching is comprehensive, effective and efficient.

One of the problems associated with helping a patient to learn about their illness, treatment and recovery is that concepts such as 'teaching' are understood in very different ways. At its simplest, teaching might consist of informing a patient about their problems and treatment. Patient information leaflets or videos might be seen as teaching materials (Sustersic et al., 2017). Typically the leaflet explains a disease in simple and accessible terms, describes the key treatment approaches and then provides contact details for further resources.

A more complex notion of teaching extends into demonstrating and explaining that required to manage an illness. So, in a case study on diabetes mellitus, those demonstrations might centre on the prevention of hypoglycaemia for example (Anuradha, 2015). Teaching in this sense requires much more interaction between the nurse and the patient, as it typically helps them to assess risk and problem-solve.

However, perhaps the most complex notion of teaching may be described as 'health coaching'. This not only addresses the cognitive (the reasoning) needs of patients but also the emotional management of sometimes lifelong challenges associated with a chronic illness. The health coach helps the patient to live with their condition, to embrace its challenges and to find new ways of thinking about themselves that seem positive. To coach is to help the patient fulfil their illness management responsibilities and it assumes the mutual identification of goals and strategies as well as criteria by which performance might be judged (O'Hara et al., 2015).

Activity 5.1   Critical thinking

Think about the three conceptions of teaching above and decide which seems to have the greatest person-centred-care potential. What do you think is involved in that form of teaching as regards the skills required of the nurse? What is entailed as regards the management of healthcare resources with that most person-centred teaching approach?

An outline answer is provided at the end of the chapter.

The conceptions of teaching briefly outlined above are often linked to different stages of the patient's illness and to their learning preferences and aptitudes (see Table 5.1). Sharing information and explaining an illness and first treatment is often associated with acute illness circumstances. While this perhaps seemed the least person-centred form of teaching, it does fit very well with the patient's acute illness circumstances. When the patient is acutely ill, perhaps an emergency admission, the capacity of the patient to learn a great deal is limited. Patients typically suffer from information overload while at the same time dealing with strange new environments (Avery et al., 2016). There is a need to understand enough to enable the patient to consent to treatment in an informed way, but they may not have mustered the confidence at this stage to collaborate more widely on future care. Patients are spending less time in hospital than in the past, so the opportunities to teach them in a more expansive way may be limited (Bergh et al., 2012). In addition to these logistical challenges, however, some patients might resist more intrusive forms of teaching, insisting that they wish to understand the facts alone and decide later how much more to investigate.

Stage of illness	Conception of teaching	Patient ability assumptions
Acute illness (something discovered and to be made sense of).	Sharing key information, informing the patient about the illness and principal treatment.	The patient can understand the information provided and appreciates what additional questions to ask.
Recovering from illness and preliminary rehabilitation.	Teaching as demonstration, explanation and question-answering.	The patient is motivated to enquire and is attentive to what is shared by the nurse. There is an exploration of the fit between clinical (risk management) and personal need.
Dealing with a chronic illness, that which the person must self-manage to a significant degree.	Health coaching.	The patient is a proactive, inquisitive and highly motivated individual who seeks to regain and retain as much control over an illness-mediated life as possible.

Table 5.1 Conceptions of teaching, stages of illness and patient ability assumptions

Teaching in the second sense, as demonstration, explanation, question and answer, the learning of skills, might operate during the recovery period in hospital, but it may well then extend into outpatient clinics, into rehabilitation programmes and perhaps into community-based support groups. By this stage the patient may well contemplate 'what next' and wish to learn skills that make them a little less dependent on healthcare staff. Indeed, a premise of much teaching in this sense is that it empowers the patient to become increasingly independent. Snow et al. (2013), for example, explains that the purpose of this teaching for diabetic patients is to enable them to become expert.

Interactive teaching represents a challenge however, and that is that it is relatively labour-intensive. In diabetes care, for example, in the DESMOND project (Developing quality Structured Education in Diabetes (Desmond Project, 2018)) learners receive six hours of teaching. In Denmark such learning may extend from a minimum of ten hours of learning to over 24 hours of teaching conducted over two to ten weeks (Laursen et al., 2017b). To make this cost-effective learning is facilitated in groups. Patients complete a course of learning that attends not only to the illness of diabetes and its successful treatment, but also to lifestyle adjustment as well, for example diet and exercise.

Not all patients learn well in large groups (Grohmann et al., 2017) and there is a growing body of knowledge relating to why patients do not attend courses (Horigan et al., 2017). Patients may drop out, fearing comparison with their peers as well as because of logistical difficulties. The debate between individual teaching with the nurse and group learning with other patients should remind you of the competing discourses that you studied in Chapter 2. The first emphasises process and individuality and the other emphasises cost-effectiveness.

Health coaching has been widely advocated as a way of helping patients to learn in a very person-centred way (Olsen, 2014). Coaching of this kind has developed apace since 2000 and it combines health education with health promotion. It combines shared goal-setting with motivational interviewing, helping the patient to identify that which might best sustain healthy behaviours. The goal of health coaching is to enlighten the individual, but also to help them to act strategically, identifying obstacles to their chosen goals and ways to overcome them. However, because the learning is so one to one, and it may extend over a protracted period of time, it is costly to deliver.

Activity 5.2   Reflecting

Think back to your own experience of learning and what seemed successful for you. Did you enjoy learning in a group and, if so, why? Did you prefer to learn privately with access to a tutor or other advisor, again, if so, why? What, when associated with an illness, might prompt you to either stick with your preferred form of learning or select another approach?

As this activity is based on your own reflection, no sample answer is provided at the end of the chapter.

Diabetes mellitus

The case study for this chapter concerns a 14-year-old boy called Tom and his mother Naomi. Tom suffers from Type 1 diabetes mellitus. Diabetes mellitus is a condition affecting the metabolism of blood glucose so that it can be utilised within cells as a source of energy, or turned into fat deposits to be stored with depot areas of the body. Sugars are derived through foodstuffs (notably carbohydrates) and rendered amenable to use by body cells through the production of insulin in the pancreas. In Type 1 diabetes mellitus the beta cells of the pancreas are progressively destroyed as part of an auto-immune response within the body. Why patients develop this form of diabetes remains unclear, but it has been postulated that both genetic and perhaps viral trigger factors play a part (Pearce, 2014). The net result of the destruction of the beta cells is that less and less insulin is available to process and reduce the level of blood sugar. Type 1 diabetes mellitus is most commonly associated with children or young adults.

Type 2 diabetes mellitus, in contrast, is not an auto-immune condition and poses a significant threat to the health of millions of people worldwide. In Canada, for example, diabetes mellitus is projected to affect 1 in 3 Canadians by the year 2020. Uncontrolled diabetes is believed to account for approximately 80 per cent of healthcare costs in Canada (Grohmann et al., 2017). The incidence of Type 1 diabetes mellitus is much less, with around 10 per cent of diagnosed cases being of this type. However, because it has onset in early life and is not open to cure, it poses a lifelong self-treatment challenge for the patient and a reliance on replacement insulin therapy.

Table 5.2 indicates the sorts of challenges that a patient diagnosed with Type 1 diabetes mellitus faces.

Problem	Notes
To control the level of dietary glucose intake (principally through controlled consumption of carbohydrates).	A patient with diabetes still needs a diet commensurate with their lifestyle energy demands/ gender, but this must be managed so as to match what subcutaneous insulin injections can help process.
To self-administer the right amount of insulin at the right times and in the right form so as to manage the level of blood glucose within target range.	Insulin is administered in different forms, short-, medium- and long-acting, in different combinations and times so as to manage the metabolic demands of the body at different times of the day and night and to match meal times when glucose intake may increase. While target blood glucose levels are agreed with the patient, it is rare for these to be achieved and sustained day in day out over the longer term (Pearce, 2014).
To re-evaluate lifestyle demands so that the right balance of glucose intake and insulin use is arrived at, adjusting the same according to periodic changes.	Young people vary their lifestyle, for example the balance of sleep and waking, time between meals, and they may make extra demands on blood glucose regulation, for instance when stressed or unwell. For that reason the balance of carbohydrate intake and insulin cannot remain a constant.
To ensure that the self-administered insulin is absorbed effectively.	The rate at which insulin is absorbed subcutaneously varies, with a slower and uneven absorption from sites used repeatedly for injection. So injection sites need to be changed. The patient might use an injection portal or an insulin pump to better regulate the supply of insulin.
To monitor for acute risks linked to an imbalance of too much insulin for too little glucose ingested (hypoglycaemia).	The most acute and potentially life-threatening risk is where a patient becomes hypoglycaemic and may collapse. Patients need to carry emergency sugar supply in the form of sweets. Patients learn to recognise early signs of hypoglycaemia.
To monitor for ongoing risks associated with inadequately controlled blood sugar levels (too much glucose in the blood) that leads to ketoacidosis, lethargia, loss of consciousness and increased risks of long-term systemic complications.	Multiple risks attend an inadequately controlled blood glucose level (hyperglycaemia), including damage to the heart, kidneys, eyes, limb circulation and brain. However, chronic, low-level hyperglycaemia may not register significantly as symptoms, making it easier for the patient to ignore that which is dangerous.
To re-evaluate self as someone who manages health in a more strategic and conscious way, managing that which did not require attention before.	Patients become people with diabetes, although in terms of owning the responsibilities for self-care they need to accept that they are diabetic. They must consciously manage their health in ways that other young people don't find a need to do.

Table 5.2   Example challenges faced by a patient diagnosed with Type 1 diabetes mellitus

Activity 5.3   Reflecting

Study Table 5.2 and note down how far-reaching the impact of Type 1 diabetes mellitus might be on a teenage boy. Remember to think of the patient as someone managing a school day, as someone who socialises and who plays sport. Some of the impact is immediate, if the patient doesn't self-care effectively he becomes ill (for instance, suffers from hypoglycaemia), but the rest of the impact is covert and accumulative (e.g., progressive damage to eyesight). What do you think the significance of this is for a patient's learning?

An outline answer is provided at the end of the chapter.

Case study: Tom and Naomi

Tom is 14. He has recently suffered from a winter viral chest infection that proved extremely difficult to overcome and he spent a period of several months feeling exhausted. He had suffered from some skin infections too and had problems concentrating on his lessons. While being investigated for these problems Tom's blood glucose levels were assessed and it was confirmed that he suffered from Type 1 diabetes mellitus. Tom has spent a short time in hospital where his blood glucose was regulated using intravenous infusions and he commenced insulin injections subcutaneously. Tom and Naomi have been given information leaflets about Type 1 diabetes mellitus and they watched a short video on the altered physiology of the condition, but now they visit the diabetes clinic of the hospital and meet Chloe, the diabetes specialist nurse.

Tom seems nervous in the clinic. In truth, the news that he has diabetes stunned him. He thought that old people got that condition. His mother, in sharp contrast, seems relieved. Naomi admits that she feared Tom might have had cancer when he started to lose weight. For Naomi now, care is all about getting down to the business of controlling what you eat and how you self-administer insulin. She has watched the nurse inject Tom with insulin. She describes the teaching already given to Tom as *instruction*, that which *Tom simply needs to learn*. Her eager approach on this, wishing to see Tom get better as quickly as possible, has been noted in Tom's care notes. Nevertheless, Tom has only tentatively taken charge of his first injections. He seems reluctant to explore further what managing diabetes entails. Chloe, the specialist nurse, runs through the things that the ward staff have already 'briefed' Tom and Naomi about. *I say briefed*, she explains to them, *because I imagine that there was a lot to take in?*

(Continued)

(Continued)

Naomi is keen to represent Tom and answers first.

No, you're right, they've told us things, showed us things haven't they Tom? We have to get on with things and do what's best for Tom's health. There is no point in fussing about this, we just have to get on with it. Tom has to give himself insulin or else he becomes very ill indeed.

Chloe wonders whether Tom feels the same. He answers,

I'm not really ready … not really. None of my mates have to do this stuff. It feels like having to have a fix. It feels like you need a needle.

Chloe nodded. Injections and illicit drugs were a common connection made by her younger patients. It had a stigma. It was something that Tom had to explain to his friends. That some form of self-care was a fait accompli, it was undeniable. In the short term he had to regulate his blood sugar effectively. In the longer term he had to avoid the complications of diabetes. Chloe smiled at Naomi. Tom's mother look understandably worried. But Chloe needed to help Tom rehearse what this meant for himself, in terms of that which he had to cope with and in terms of ways in which he might learn. She said to Tom,

You can't be expected to learn everything in a day. Your friends can't demand everything explained in an instant. You have time to learn and time to get better looking after yourself. I was wondering what you think you have to learn Tom?

Tom summarised what he could remember from the hospital ward. He had to manage his carbohydrate intake, food like potatoes. He had to think again about sugary drinks. Tom continued, explaining that, normally, inside you, there was something near your stomach that made insulin and it was this in your blood that converted food to sugar for your muscles. As he didn't produce much of that, he had to have injections and to learn to give them to himself.

Chloe wanted to know what he noticed about symptoms? What did having diabetes feel like in terms of being unwell?

When I was sick, I seemed to sleep all the time. I seemed unable to do much at all. I got headaches and I felt like I would never play football again.

She asked what he might feel if the opposite happened, if he had too much insulin, perhaps by mistake, if he gave himself too much?

They said that I'd get dizzy and flake out. I could injure myself.

Yes, said Chloe. She explained to Tom that there were some different things to learn, but the first things that she could teach him were concerned with what he felt, the symptoms. If she dealt with those and what could happen, then she hoped that he might feel safer? Some of the other learning, to do with how diabetes could be a problem over many years, might be built up later on. She asked whether that seemed reasonable to him.

I don't want to flake out. I don't want to have an accident. I don't want to look sick, you know, like I'm having a fit or something. Tom said.

So we can talk a bit about food, about injections and about checking the sugar in your blood. We can talk about you getting on with things in your own way, for now, in these next days. We can start to control what you've found tiring, worrying? Chloe smiled.

Tom checked his mother's face, and then he nodded at Chloe.

We can set the more technical things aside for the weeks ahead. There are some expert things, some things that might help you feel good about yourself and help you deal with your friends, the teachers, may be a doctor when you see one?

Tom nodded again.

I'm an arts kid, I'm not doing sciences at school. I'm not a maths wizard or anything. Drugs, mixing them up, that scares me, he explained.

So we should start there and keep it simple, suggested Chloe, *then we can go on later to why things happen as they do, how you can head off long-term problems. I wondered, how do you like learning at school?*

Tom thought for a moment or two.

I like learning the facts first and then going back, in a tutorial, to check that I have them straight. I like my tutor in English, he makes the explanations fun. He doesn't smirk if I describe things wrong.

Chloe nodded.

One of the ways in which some people learn about diabetes is by going on a short course. It's just a couple of afternoons, around six or seven hours. But it's a mix of people, different ages. How might that seem?

Tom grimaced.

Don't want to look stupid. I don't do role play or anything like that!

Chloe laughed.

No role play, but the people who go on those courses, some of them are older. Diabetes, it affects people at different ages. You know? she ventured.

Tom thought that would seem *strange,* may be *freaky.*

Chloe thought again. While some courses might be run for teenagers alone, most she knew about involved patients of different ages and backgrounds.

What about something else. I know a girl called Gina, she's eighteen and has been looking after her diabetes for almost two years. She had a few problems, around her exams, so she came back to

(Continued)

(Continued)

see me and we spent some time going over things again. She said that helped and that she'd help me with other people with diabetes. I've another patient called Toby who I help. I was thinking of forming a tutorial group that maybe you could help us make up. What do you think?

Naomi nodded enthusiastically, but Chloe's attention was fixed on Tom. She waited. Naomi started to talk, but Chloe gently touched her hand and her gaze returned once more to Tom.

Yes, that sound's good, I'd like to try it that way, he said.

Activity 5.4   Critical thinking

Look back at the case study above and then answer the following questions.

1.   Why do you think Chloe invited Tom to describe the learning challenges in his own words?
2.   Why do you think it important that she emphasised that learning could be incremental?
3.   What do you think was the rationale of planning teaching first that centred on symptoms, that which had happened and that might happen?
4.   What within this dialogue suggests that she is thinking very hard and considerately about Tom's needs?

As this activity is based on your own reflection, no sample answer is provided at the end of the chapter.

Anticipating the needs and concerns of the patient

The primary source of ideas for person-centred care that Chloe drew upon was her case study patient Gina. Gina's teenage years were chaotic. She suffered from gluten intolerance that made her diet more complex and that meant that the amount of glucose that she absorbed from meals seemed to vary markedly. Whatever calculation Gina learned about matching insulin to food intake barely seemed to work. The problem was that not only did Gina's blood glucose levels seem to swing alarmingly back and forth, but also that she then compounded that with a weight control regimen that she tried to run while preparing for examinations. The wish to feel in control loomed large in Gina's mind and it wasn't centred solely on blood glucose levels as clinical risk policies encouraged.

What profoundly impressed Chloe, though, was what Gina taught her about a young person's psychology. The need to control self, to control image was very important. That which attended to image control, to the management of what might happen, might well appear as most needful to other teenage patients as well. As you can't routinely see diabetes, then the teenager's attention often focussed on keeping it that way, off radar. Gina had presented Chloe with lots of challenges, but she was an articulate patient. There was every likelihood that she might help Tom. A small 'tutorial' group that met with Chloe and Gina every month might be a good way to further problem-solving teaching over the year ahead.

Teaching patients with diabetes

In many regards the ideal support relationship for a teenager was a health coaching one. Chloe had read O'Hara et al.'s (2015) work on health coaching and noted that this could be done by telephone. It was especially powerful because it not only attended to barriers that patients had to overcome, but also because it set up a framework for monitoring patient progress. Of all the teaching approaches there are, health coaching attended best to the emotional management of diabetes. Health coaching could help counter anxiety, depression, frustrations with treatment and also help to sustain self-esteem. However, the problem was that Chloe's patient caseload was too great to offer such help. Therefore, working with a more experienced patient seemed a reasonable compromise. Small-group teaching was more cost-efficient than one-to-one teaching.

NHS England (2018) describe this period in the patient's recovery and adjustment as the patient activation period. During this time it was important for Chloe to start building the patient's knowledge, their skills and their confidence. The goal of her support, then, was to start moving Tom to a state where he had enough confidence to start managing his own health. That which helped activate a patient was usually that which seemed closest to their experience of problems. Motivation was driven by experience of threat or discomfort, not by a more abstract discussion of diabetes mellitus as a condition.

Reviewing the alternative of asking Tom to enrol on a course, Chloe noted the following.

- To be effective, courses needed a clear structure and to focus on healthy lifestyle as well as illness management (Snow et al., 2013; McDowell and MacRury, 2015; Laursen et al., 2017a).
- Courses could cause performance anxiety, however, as patients compared their mastery of treatment with that of others (Laursen et al., 2017a).
- Against that, group-learning courses could seem liberating as patients felt that they achieved a more rounded explanation of why the condition affected them as it did (Snow et al., 2013). For the more confident patient, group-learning taught them the 'tools of the trade' that they might need in future consultations with medical staff.

In their study of locating patient education services for diabetic patients within the primary care area, Grohmann et al. (2017) observed that the relocation of service overcame some of the problems that patients experienced in persevering with courses. By moving education closer to the patient and frequently working with smaller groups, nurses were able to offer more individual support.

Hearing the patient narrative and identifying possible ways forward

Listening to Tom was important to Chloe. However much she respected and valued the contribution of Naomi, in the longer term it would be Tom who had to manage his illness. Managing diabetes, in Chloe's experience, was intimately to do with what diabetes meant to the individual patient. So, in the consultation, Chloe consciously and politely focussed on Tom's first reasoning. Afterwards, when Tom visited the toilet, Chloe explained the reasoning of this to Naomi. Both son and mother were Chloe's clients, both had a vested interest in the service that she offered, but there was a need to quickly establish how Tom thought about his problem and how he might wish to go about solving it in the future. Chloe put it this way to Naomi,

Sometimes, there's a risk that we want to solve a patient's problems for them, to help them perfect something as fast as we can. That would be my instinct, as a parent, to protect. But I've found that we need to understand how teenagers are thinking about a problem as well. My dad, he knew how to do something really well and when I was trying to make something, in woodwork, he would show me again and again. I gave up on the woodwork, because he didn't let me work much out for myself. I remember, the woodwork project got finished, but I never went back and did another with him.

Activity 5.5   Reflecting

Care for children and young people is designed to be family-centred, acknowledging the interplay of roles between parents and children and between siblings. So pause now to reflect on how well you think Chloe is doing working with Naomi as Tom begins his work on learning to self-care. There is a risk that an established carer is affronted by the contribution of a new carer. Do you think that Chloe seems alert to this? How important is it that Chloe explains her strategy to Naomi?

An outline answer is provided at the end of the chapter.

In this consultation Chloe believed that Tom understood the rudiments of diabetes mellitus as a glucose-processing problem, although he lacked any insights into the challenges of finding the balance between food intake, blood glucose levels and the planned insulin to be injected at carefully timed intervals. Tom understood the basic problem, but he had little understanding of illness management. He didn't understand how food and insulin imbalance might create signs and symptoms that could worry him.

What interested Chloe specifically, however, was the level of confidence that Tom showed in overcoming the challenges that he now faced. There was a risk through well-meant parental enthusiasm that mother and child might simply assert that 'we will beat this thing'. Understanding Tom's confidence levels was critical as low levels of confidence might undermine the teaching she offered. Simply layering on more information, showing more about how to do things (skills), risked overwhelming Tom.

Whatever the service imperative to teach and discharge to the care of others, there was a need to work with what Tom felt he could learn. It was for that reason that Chloe listened attentively to how Tom described his problem. She noticed the analogy that Tom made when describing someone who had fainted from hypoglycaemia. It might look like a fit. In Chloe's experience such problems were disturbing for teenagers. The sudden loss of control, without explanation, represented a significant possible loss of face. What might therefore motivate Tom? A fear of lost control, disturbing self-image, might be the driver that she could use to help him focus on the importance of managing his insulin injections, at the right dose and at the right time.

Moving things forward

In moving to exploring possible ways for Tom to learn, Chloe had no strategic plan to build a tutorial group. She was aware of regional courses available to help patients learn a great deal more about successfully managing diabetes mellitus. Importantly, such courses enabled parents of young patients to join in. But what did seem to be an issue for Tom was that they had both an age range of patients and operated in comparatively larger groups. While such a course might still benefit Tom later on, the early confidence-building work that Tom needed seemed better suited to a more intimate environment. It was routine that over the next months Chloe would teach Tom some key skills and answer his questions in clinic, but it was the business of thinking more widely about control that seemed amenable to a small group solution.

Chloe freely admitted that, at this stage, she was speculating about what might be successful. She already knew a great deal about Gina and about Toby and she was sure that they would be amenable to some group meetings, but she had not originally conceived of these as tutorials. What struck Chloe was that some forms of learning were already familiar and seemed supportive to Tom. Toby, too, was attending secondary education so he also might be familiar with tutorials. It seemed possible, then, that structuring health learning in terms of other learning already familiar to Tom might have a greater chance of success.

Activity 5.6   Speculating

Pause now to think about Chloe's plan to arrange some of the teaching within a tutorial group format. This has the potential to reduce the number of times she needs to teach things to different patients. But what do you think of it as an innovation? Does it surprise you that person-centred care is not always one to one?

An outline answer is provided at the end of the chapter.

Person-centred care insights

By the time you finished reading the third case study of this book you may have been struck by just how important nurse expertise is. Each of the nurses involved in the care of the three patients introduced in case studies so far has a significant fund of experience to draw upon, each is keenly aware of relevant research evidence and each has developed some confidence in reasoning how best to mix experience and evidence together. It is certainly true that it is only as the nurse develops familiarity with a field of healthcare practice, and with a well-understood population of patients, that they can deliver care that seems both expert and person-centred.

Adopting the right attitude

But even without such expertise something can quickly be identified with regard to what may be necessary when approaching patients. This relates to attitude. It is unrealistic to provide patients with all that they might hope to receive, all that they might believe that they need. Not every patient or lay carer perception is wise. Patients might demand things that could place them at significant risk, things based on misunderstanding of a disease or treatment. But it is possible to help patients and lay carers to attend very carefully to the experience of illness, treatment and care in ways that enable them to achieve increasing independence. In the case study of Tom, it would be comparatively easy to simply accede to the felt need of a carer, especially a parent. The felt need to resolve a difficulty, to counter a threat, is part of feeling protective. Naomi told Chloe that she imagined that they would briskly move on to more skills. She hadn't thought about how that teaching would be arranged, but she guessed that *there was a plan for this.*

It is a natural instinct to want to solve the problem as quickly as possible, but wisdom in this instance balances the meeting of a felt need with insights from elsewhere to recommend something to Tom. Care is not necessarily served by teaching the patient as many skills as possible, as quickly as possible (Snow et al., 2013). In delivering person-centred care the nurse does not surrender expertise, but she still uses it sensitively and strategically.

Reviewing the standard solution

In this case study Chloe considers what she already knows about course learning for patients with diabetes. There is a growing body of evidence about the merits and the limits of course learning. Course learning is widely advocated, but there remain some concerns about its success. Little has been discussed with regard to the age of the learner, different levels of learning ability and the suitability of course-based learning. If people learn in different ways at different stages of their lives, can the common experience of an illness circumvent that and enable them all to learn together? On this occasion the more powerful influence on Chloe's thinking has been a familiar case study. Gina has had a profound effect on Chloe's assessment of how younger patients learn. She has been persuaded that the mistakes that Gina made, the problems that she has overcome, may have a great deal to offer Tom.

Working with patient perceptions

In this consultation Chloe started by asking Tom to describe his illness in his own terms. Chloe's approach has a number of pragmatic purposes. The first is that Tom's summary helps her to understand how much he appears to know. But as equally important as whether Tom's understanding is accurate or not is how he describes the problem, what he focusses on most. Tom's emphasis on mishaps, accidents, untoward events such as collapsing when hypoglycaemic suggests to Chloe what she might use to motivate Tom's learning. She will certainly need to teach Tom about blood glucose monitoring and judging the right dose of insulin to self-administer, but what will reinforce that learning is what he can avoid more effectively by getting the calculations right.

Prioritising teaching

Chloe also emphasises that learning could be incremental. In person-centred care it is important to carefully consider the workload that patients are asked to shoulder. Chronic illnesses such as diabetes mellitus load patients with new self-care responsibilities. A large amount of new responsibility might overwhelm a patient and make it much harder for them to believe that they can succeed. So, in this instance, when the patient lacks confidence, it is important to remind them that learning is done over time and that the nurse is there to help them to prioritise what they learn first. More abstract threats associated with damage to body organs associated with prolonged hyperglycaemia will need to be attended to as well, but the first work is with patient safety and that which Tom already knows about, i.e., what it is like to experience symptoms of illness.

Chloe is thinking very hard about Tom's needs. She is thinking reflexively, that is, she is thinking about what Tom is telling her, but also about how her suggestions seem to resonate for him. Chloe demonstrates considerable interest in Tom's needs by asking him about how he sees his problem, how he experiences the illness. She is willing to speculate with him about the learning that might best assist him. This could seem an unusual question to ask a patient. After all, it is more comfortable and familiar for the nurse to use a standard way to address the learning that patients have to complete. They may concentrate on what they know must be taught and less on how it might be learned. In person-centred care, though, the two must be blended. Giving information alone is not the entirety of teaching, you need to assist the patient in what sense they make of the information and to establish why it is worth knowing.

Chapter summary

In this chapter we have explored the relationship between teaching and person-centred care. In many ways it highlights a recurring challenge within person-centred care, that is, initially, the nurse often knows a great deal more about a condition than the patient does. Later, in chronic illnesses, this imbalance of understanding and knowledge may be reversed as the patient becomes expert. But, for now, to facilitate the patient's learning involves a few niceties of judgement.

- It is important to understand that teaching might be thought of in different ways and that patients might hope that you will teach them in ways that seem familiar and comfortable.
- Teaching may change in format over the passage of time; it may, for instance, become group-based rather than individual-based. Learning in a group may suit some patients very well indeed but you should not assume that this is always the case.
- What the nurse hopes to teach (clinical need) and what the patient hopes to learn (felt need) might not be quite the same thing. Therefore, in order to reinforce rapport with the patient, the nurse must clearly attend to felt need issues early on.
- Learning to cope with an illness usually involves an emotional component and here there is significant scope for the nurse to demonstrate a truly person-centred care. In this case study example, Tom is especially sensitive to how having diabetes mellitus might seem to his friends and what it might look like if he suffers a hypoglycaemic attack. Chloe uses that understanding to focus her early teaching with him.

Activities: Brief outline answers

Activity 5.1   Critical thinking (p87)

I wonder if you agree with me that health coaching seems the most intrinsically person-centred, but also potentially the most labour-intensive? Simply providing information and explanations seems the least person-centred as information is often presented in an unimaginative way. Whether health coaching represents an excellent if initially costly investment depends on whether it subsequently obviates the need for future problem-solving treatment and care. This is difficult to assess as investment costs and rewards are borne by different parts of the healthcare service, perhaps funded from different sources. The return on a coaching investment may come over several decades ahead.

Activity 5.3   Reflecting (p91)

The impact of diabetes mellitus is far-reaching for a teenage boy, largely because, while hidden (the individual might not look diabetic), it affects many of the lifestyle freedoms that are frequently associated with youth. So, for example, a teenage boy might frequently change his sleep/wake pattern, staying up late into the night and catching up with sleep at the weekends. But the pattern of sleeping and wakefulness affects appetite and the utilisation of glucose. When the body clock shifts we may eat more carbohydrates, especially convenience food. This poses problems for managing the insulin regimen. The implications of this for patient learning may be that Tom has to consider how much of his lifestyle can or should be varied, when penalties may accrue with regard to maintenance of an acceptable blood glucose level. Compromises may have to be sought between lifestyle and the complication risks of diabetes if blood glucose is not controlled.

Activity 5.5   Reflecting (p96)

If you regularly work with parents of sick children or young people you may have already experienced the delicate negotiation of care responsibilities and authority that can ensue. It is by no means easy for lay carers and nurses to partner in care. Chloe needs to remain alert to how her questions and recommendations seem to a parent. Nevertheless, in this instance, the expertise of the nurse offered to Naomi and Tom relates not only to diabetes, but also to the business of learning self-care. However urgently a parent might wish for the nurse to get on with doing something for the patient, there is a need to focus too on how confident Tom feels and how he thinks he learns best. Chloe knows that understanding this well may determine how successful Tom's learning is, so she must make the expert point to Naomi. The anxiety-reduction needs of a parent may not exactly coincide with the learning needs of a sick young person.

Activity 5.6   Speculating (p98)

In Chapter 2 the case was made that pragmatic person-centred care was often locally innovative. It grew not out of a formula for care but out of speculation about what might work well for individual patients. In this instance, Chloe doesn't know yet what the challenges of running a tutorial group will be, but she is confident that Gina can help Tom to learn about managing diabetes and his treatment. Sometimes the most person-centred care involves thinking out of the box. Chloe can defend this initiative as she will secure permissions from all patients and guardians concerned, and because she can demonstrate that there are also service savings associated with teaching that might otherwise have to be one to one for both Toby and Tom.

Further reading

A debate continues within healthcare services across the world about the best ways to educate patients about their illness and self-care treatment. On the one hand, education work could be assigned to specialist teams and much more use might be made of courses to educate groups of patients. On the other hand, education might remain intrinsic to the work of many healthcare professionals who meet patients in clinics, wards, the home and surgeries. Both of the following textbooks offer a comprehensive review of the sorts of things that nurses and others might teach. For any of you eager to engage in such future work these texts are useful places to start.

Bastable, S (2016) *Essentials of Patient Education,* 2nd edition. London: Jones and Barkett Publishers.

Mertig, R (2012) *Nurses' Guide to Teaching Patients Self Management,* 2nd edition. New York: Springer.

Useful websites

An interesting exercise to do is to visit several websites that offer teaching on the management of a condition. It is then possible to assess to what extent they seem person-centred. That is, does the site seem to acknowledge the diversity of individuals' experiences and needs? Does it respect the emotional dimension of coping with an illness? Is there scope for the patient/individual to actively engage with the teaching presented in some way? Below are some sample teaching websites that I hope will be of interest to nurses working in different fields of healthcare practice.

www.diabetes.co.uk/how-to/control-diabetes.html

How to control diabetes – foods, diet, blood testing and motivation.

www.moodjuice.Scot.nhs.uk/anxiety.asp

MOODJUICE – anxiety self-help guide.

www.autism.org.uk>Professionals>Employers>Information_for_employers

Managing an autistic employee – NAS.

Chapter 6 Helping patients to rehabilitate

NMC Standards of Proficiency for Registered Nurses

This chapter will address the following platforms and proficiencies:

Platform 1: Being an accountable professional

At the point of registration, the registered nurse will be able to:

1.8 demonstrate the knowledge, skills and ability to think critically when applying evidence and drawing on experience to make evidence informed decisions in all situations.

1.9 understand the need to base all decisions regarding care and interventions on people's needs and preferences, recognising and addressing any personal and external factors that may unduly influence your decisions.

Chapter aims

After reading this chapter, you will be able to:

- understand the ways in which person-centred care might be demonstrated as part of patient rehabilitation;
- understand the requirement for practitioners to 'think again' about their practice assumptions, finding innovative ways to attend to need and to revise service.

Introduction

So much of what makes person-centred care successful and practical relies on the three-way interaction of evidence, experience and adequately listened-to patient narrative. In Chapter 2 of this book I located evidence within the 'anticipating patient needs' work of the nurse. That can seem as though evidence always precedes interactive care work with the patient. In practice, however, the different sorts of work interact more fluently than that and it is sometimes the case that needs and concerns identified with a patient prompt the search for different kinds of evidence, or else the memory of evidence elsewhere, that could work. The ability to manage care in this way constitutes the nous (the common-sense thinking) of the nurse.

Once a patient has successfully completed their recovery from an illness or injury, many will move into a period of rehabilitation. Rehabilitation is necessary where the patient requires further help in order to manage their ongoing lives (Slomic et al., 2016). The purpose of rehabilitation is to:

- sustain the improvements in the patient's health (for example, by teaching patients how to use medications);
- to further the patient's independence and capacity to adapt to ongoing challenges (for example, through exercise regimes);
- to develop self-belief so that the patient becomes proactive in care deliberations (for example, through patient counselling).

Rehabilitation work with patients affords nurses an excellent opportunity to practice person-centred care. This is because there are longer periods of time over which the nurse–patient professional relationship can grow. To rehabilitate successfully, patients usually need to think afresh about their circumstances and to find new ways of conceiving of themselves and their lifestyle (Ghisi et al., 2015). While the precise focus and format of rehabilitation may vary between different specialist areas of practice, there are common denominators between all areas. Patients have to take stock of the challenges before them, to reconsider issues associated with risk and to evaluate what adjustments in living may be necessary. Patients may increase their knowledge base associated with a problem, develop new skills and engage closely with others to ascertain what progress is being made. Irrespective of whether patients are rehabilitating within the areas of physical health, mental health, child health and wellbeing, care of the older person or of those with intellectual disabilities, patients are embarked upon a learning journey (Tiller et al., 2013).

Activity 6.1 Reflecting

Think back to a patient that you have helped to rehabilitate. Which of the above purposes of rehabilitation featured most strongly and why?

An outline answer is provided at the end of the chapter.

Cardiac rehabilitation, that recommended after an acute myocardial infarction (a 'heart attack'), represents an excellent test area for person-centred care. This is because, in the first instance, the patient suffers a sudden and often a frightening change in their health status (Wlodarcyzk, 2017). Not all patients suffer the classic gripping chest pain described in cardiology textbooks. Some patients might encounter much less dramatic symptoms, a shortness of breath, feelings of dyspepsia and perhaps faintness (Whittaker et al., 2012). However, all patients will at some point undergo an electrocardiogram (ECG) and will have been informed that they have suffered a 'heart attack'.

The first 20–40 minutes of the heart attack are vital as it is in this period of time that irreversible damage starts to occur to that proximal portion of the myocardium (heart muscle) served by the blocked coronary artery (Kulick, 2018). Prompt treatment, in the form of coronary angiography (the visualisation of the coronary arteries using a catheter from a distal blood vessel) and the introduction of a stent (a mesh insert to hold a stretched artery open so that blood flows through), is usually the preferred treatment. More patients survive heart attacks as a result of prompt invasive treatment but there then remains a residue of rehabilitation work to complete regarding that which contributed to the problem in the first place:

- lack of exercise;
- genetic predisposition to atheroma formation in the blood vessels (high levels of cholesterol);
- high blood pressure;
- and a diet high in fats.

Patients have to begin to exercise their hearts once again so that the remaining muscle power is used most effectively (Abell et al., 2015).

Activity 6.2   Reflecting

Review how you and your colleagues, prior to nurse training, conceived of the heart. For example, did you think of it as a clock or battery? Patients sometimes refer to their hearts as their 'ticker'. Did you conceive of it as a pump, something that pushed blood around the body?

An outline answer is provided at the end of the chapter.

Nurses assisting post-myocardial-infarction patients to rehabilitate are closely involved with several of the sorts of work that you were introduced to in Chapter 2. The nurse must utilise relevant evidence, listen carefully to the patient's narrative and identify ways forward with the patient as part of the rehabilitation plan. But they must also determine with the patient, and often with their partner, what counts as rehabilitation progress and the parts that are most usefully played by supporters. Patients undergoing cardiac rehabilitation rapidly accumulate experiences, both good and bad, and it is then vital that the nurse learns from these in order to recommend adjustments to the mutually agreed care plan (Ghisi et al., 2015). In this chapter's case study I introduce you to Roy, a 45-year-old man who has suffered a myocardial infarct, with no prior history of angina. As you will see, Roy has significant misgivings about his rehabilitation and that brings him into conflict with his wife.

Case study: Roy

Invited to describe himself to you, Roy would say that he is middle-aged and has probably spent more time watching football than playing it. Much of his working life has been spent in moving pallets of goods around a warehouse on a forklift truck. Roy is married to Joan and they lead a simple life, watching spectator sports, eating fish and chips on a Friday night and having a few drinks at the pub. Roy is clinically obese. He has given up cigarette smoking because his brother Phil was diagnosed with emphysema, raised blood cholesterol and was commenced on statins to reduce the risks to his heart.

Seven weeks ago Roy began to experience some symptoms that he linked to work. He felt exhausted and he was quickly breathless. He suffered some pain in his neck and jaw, which came on suddenly. He told Joan about his experiences and said that he might now visit their GP. Joan, though, dismissed the problem and said that men made a fuss about very minor problems. He should give it a few weeks to see whether it settled. Then, four weeks ago, Roy felt giddy and he fell to the floor, struggling for breath. He had a pain in his lower chest and Joan summoned an ambulance. An ECG was completed and Roy was told that he was suffering a heart attack. It was necessary to go to theatre where a catheter would be inserted into his leg and fed up into his left coronary artery to unblock a clot that had formed there. The surgeon would stretch his blood vessel using a balloon on the catheter tip and then put in a stent, something that would ensure blood flow was restored to the damaged muscle (Khan, 2018).

The operation was successful, although Roy described it as 'a bit of a drama'. Joan was mortified because she had dissuaded him from visiting the doctor. Roy had to start medication to support his damaged heart. He would take a low dose of aspirin daily to reduce the stickiness of blood platelets that could risk another coronary artery blockage. He was to take a beta blocker to help reduce his rapid heart rate (atenolol). He was also to start a statin drug similar to that taken by his brother (simvastatin). This drug was designed to reduce the production of cholesterol within the liver, that which risked forming new atheroma in his arteries.

Once the doctors had assessed his progress, Roy was recommended to join an eight-week cardiac rehabilitation programme run at the hospital. The nurse co-ordinator for that was called Alicia and she visited Roy to describe what it entailed. First there would be a carefully calibrated aerobic exercise programme, one that worked within his own tolerance levels. The circuit training sessions would involve a carefully managed warm-up and a wind-down session either side of the 20 or so minutes of exercise. A physiotherapist was on hand to guide Roy. The programme also included teaching about a healthy diet, exercise planning and some relaxation sessions that were designed to help Roy counter the stress in his life.

Roy was very anxious about the rehabilitation programme as he worried that it might trigger another heart attack. He had imagined that rest rather than exercise was what would heal his heart. Joan, however, was desperately keen that he did attend and achieved the necessary change in lifestyle. Reluctantly, Roy commenced the programme. In the third week of the programme a new acquaintance of Roy's (William) suffered a cardiac arrest and staff were unsuccessful in resuscitating him. The heart attack had happened as he started his own exercise session on a day that Roy was attending. Roy was devastated and point-blank refused to continue. Joan shouted at him that he must continue and came immediately to Alicia, asking her to reinforce the message that Roy must continue regardless.

Activity 6.3   Critical thinking

Before reading on, jot down what you think the key problems for Roy and his wife are at this stage. Why do you think it is vital that Alicia attends closely to the narratives involved as well as to any evidence that she may have accrued?

An outline answer is provided at the end of the chapter.

Attending to the needs and concerns of the patient

While Alicia had significant evidence relating to cardiac rehabilitation, relatively little of it was to do with sustaining patients as they completed their programmes. Still, she was sure that a consensus opinion among her clinical colleagues had something new to offer for the care that they delivered. So powerful was this 'hunch' about psychology and care that she had proposed some qualitative research that would begin soon. The work focussed on patient conceptions of the heart and the influence that this might have on their success engaging with the exercise programme. Colleagues speculated that patients tended to conceive of the heart either as a battery or as a pump. Those that saw the heart as a battery might fear the inevitable failure of the heart, while those who conceived of it as a pump might envisage repairs. Conceptions of the heart might then shape patient response to rehabilitation.

As Alicia listened to Joan's concerns about her husband's planned withdrawal from the cardiac rehabilitation programme, Alicia wondered how he thought about his heart? In addition to local speculation about patient psychology, Alicia could point to a couple of studies that described barriers to successful rehabilitation.

- Williams et al. (2011) described a D-type personality that struggled to adopt and sustain recommended cardiac medications post-heart attack. Type D individuals were very prone to anxiety and they were not openly expressive of their problems.
- Figueiras et al. (2017) had reviewed just how important cardiac misconceptions were among patients following acute myocardial infarction. They argued that their correction as part of the plan of care had a material impact post-heart attack on patient levels of exercise, smoking, the return to work and patient mood. Rehabilitation work had to correct misconceptions such as that the heart muscle could not be strengthened.

A problem presented itself as regards the evidence-based literature, that which patients and their families sometimes read online. The evidence for the effectiveness of cardiac rehabilitation remained ambiguous (see Table 6.1). The problem for Alicia was that if a patient cited the literature to her, she couldn't honestly claim that there were unambiguous outcome benefits associated with completing rehabilitation programmes.

Authors in favour of cardiac rehabilitation programmes	Authors critical of cardiac rehabilitation programmes
• Cardiac rehabilitation limits cardiac mortality, forestalling additional infarctions (Heran et al., 2011). • Rehabilitation helps limit the health problems attendant on poorer perfusion of the myocardium (morbidity) (Anderson et al., 2016).	• Lifestyle adjustments best carried out before patients suffer a heart attack (Forman, 2016). • Patients completing cardiac rehabilitation programmes secure no significant long-term benefits over others who don't (West et al., 2012).

Table 6.1 Different assessments of cardiac rehabilitation programmes

Nevertheless, it was possible to assert that cardiac rehabilitation still represented a good investment. Cardiac rehabilitation improved quality of life for targeted patients and in a cost-efficient way in the UK (Moghei et al., 2017). It was possible to arrange such programmes in different ways, for instance in locations away from the hospital (Schopfer and Forman, 2016; Clark et al., 2015).

Activity 6.4   Speculating

How do you think that the 'mixed messages' research literature might be used by a patient to either embrace or reject a cardiac rehabilitation programme? If you were Alicia, how might you represent evidence to a patient such as Roy so that he can better evaluate whether or not to withdraw from the programme he enrolled upon?

An outline answer is provided at the end of the chapter.

Hearing the patient narrative and identifying possible ways forward

Much as Alicia would have liked the research evidence to be unambiguous and to answer all of Joan and Roy's concerns, in this instance it seemed unequal to the task in hand. A variety of problems attend evidence-based care:

- The evidence may be contradictory (as in this case);
- it may be fragmented (perhaps dealing with different populations of patients);
- or it might offer little contextual fit (for instance, treatments may have advanced and changed since the research was done).

The fact that Alicia and her colleagues were planning new research highlights the current evidence uncertainty. In person-centred care, practitioners are willing to carefully speculate on what might be happening and needed, and to plan research accordingly.

Patient and lay carer narratives

In this case study Alicia had two narratives to consider. The first and most important one was that of Roy. Alicia had to learn from Roy's experiences, his insights and fears, in order to advise him about what to decide regarding whether or not to continue with the programme. The second important narrative was that of Joan. Joan felt guilty about not encouraging Roy to request help earlier in his illness. Her enthusiasm for the programme could be motivated both by personal guilt and by fear for Roy's health in the future.

Still, Alicia was aware that patients frequently delayed seeking medical help in the face of cardiac symptoms. This could be influenced by a variety of factors: the context in which the events occurred (did symptoms accumulate slowly for example), symptomatology (some signs of cardiac decline ran silent, there was not always chest pain for instance) and lay advice from others (Roy might have received other counsel beyond Joan's that symptoms frequently 'blow over') (Coventry et al., 2017). Care in this case had to be delivered both to Roy and to Joan. If the couple did not receive what seemed wise counsel, then they might negatively evaluate the service in the weeks ahead.

Joan's narrative

Alicia listened to Joan's account of events. Joan recounted in florid detail how she had dismissed Roy's growing concerns. She explained that now, when another patient had died, Roy was becoming so risk-adverse that the very thing that he feared might come to pass precisely because he failed to exercise his heart. Roy sat in the chair too much, he ate too many take-away meals and he drank too much beer. She admitted that they were both overweight. Here is an extract from how she summarised this.

> *I feel as if we're a disaster waiting to happen Alicia. I've fed him the wrong food, I've encouraged the wrong habits and then I went and ignored his problems when he described them to me. We've been complacent. Roy is only in his forties. We should live into our eighties shouldn't we? That's what the newspapers say. If we go on living this way we'll be lucky to make it to 60!*

Alicia heard regret, fear and guilt together in Joan's explanation. Joan felt that she was to blame for her husband's newly discovered risks. Now that Roy was planning to withdraw from the programme, Joan saw that risk increasing rapidly. But Alicia had some questions regarding what Joan was saying. Did she see the rehabilitation programme as a quick-fix solution, that which was time-critical now, or did she see it as one aid to lifestyle change, that which required attention for the rest of their lives? There was a risk that Joan assumed the hospital-based programme was the best, perhaps the only programme.

Alicia: *Tell me about the programme and how you see that working Joan.*

Joan: *Well, it's another sort of treatment. As I see it, Roy's refusing treatment and that makes me so angry and so frightened. It's as if he thinks his stent can do all the work for him!*

Alicia: *A stent helps a great deal, but Roy has other arteries in his heart and they don't have stents fitted.*

Joan: *Exactly! You should tell him that. You should tell him to finish the programme otherwise he could die early.*

Alicia: *Can the rehabilitation programme guarantee to Roy that he will add a lot of years to his life do you think?*

Joan: *Nothing is guaranteed, I know that Alicia.*

Alicia: *So Roy is speculating. He's making an investment and there is a reasonable chance that benefits can accrue if he changes his lifestyle and loses some weight. But other risk factors, his high cholesterol levels, we can modify those but we can't remove them.*

Joan: *No we can't, I know. But I want him to try. I want him to at least have a go.*

As Alicia listened to Joan she was reminded of two other papers she had read.

Helping patients sustain hope

The first paper had been written by Wlodarcyzk (2017) and that concerned optimism and hope among post-myocardial infarction patients. The paper argued that social support and a problem-solving attitude were both important to post-heart attack patients. Patients needed to hope that they could recover and then they had to have faith in the measures that they used to adjust their lives for the future (optimism). It was important that Roy and Joan tackled this problem together. So, whatever Roy and Joan finally agreed to do, the next steps that they took needed to seem hopeful and to offer reasons why rehabilitation seemed beneficial. Living post-myocardial infarction was not really about statistics, it was about feeling coherent, purposeful, doing something that recognised what had happened, but that facilitated living tolerably with anxiety as well.

Countering fatigue, assessing risk

The second paper that Alicia suddenly remembered concerned fatigue (Alsen and Eriksson, 2016). These authors reported just how prominent fatigue was among post-myocardial infarction patients and how distressing it was. The problem was that all people felt fatigued at one time or another, but that fatigue posed a particular worry for the patient after a heart attack. Fatigue might be the precursor of another collapse. What Joan and possibly Roy really required was not so much a guarantee that the rehabilitation 'would work', but that efforts there, plus some better personal monitoring, might help them to assess risk over the months ahead.

Alicia wondered whether the programme that she coordinated addressed personal monitoring that well. Apart from the aerobic exercise regimen, the lifestyle guidance centred on better eating and exercising and on stress reduction exercises. It seemed to Alicia that it consisted of patching activities. It centred on corrective and prescriptive measures. There was relatively little on reading health afterwards. Targets (weight, waist measurements, blood cholesterol levels) were not the same thing as attending to experiences. It was easier to focus on signs, as those seemed scientific. Attending to symptoms tended to emphasise fear.

Activity 6.5   Critical thinking

What do you notice about the interplay of evidence and listened-to narrative as Alicia explores problems with Joan? Does one or other seem more important? Is there a way in which combining narrative insights with evidence might assist Alicia to overcome her own frustration with the ambiguous outcomes attributed to cardiac rehabilitation programmes?

An outline answer is provided at the end of the chapter.

Alicia explained to Joan that the cardiac rehabilitation programmes were reported in the literature as achieving mixed outcomes. She briefly outlined why researchers could reach different conclusions. However, she also suggested that it was probably more important that the programme was seen as their tool rather than a 'treatment'. No programme lasting a number of weeks could inoculate the patient against risk. Whether or not Roy suffered another heart attack depended on what he did with the teaching and the coping responses taught to him.

A programme of this kind was not a one-time opportunity; it was possible to enrol upon a programme later and one perhaps based closer to their home. While withdrawal from the programme might be ill-considered, it wasn't an irrevocable decision. There were other opportunities to explore later if they wished to do so. Alicia promised to talk with Roy about his concerns later that day. In the interim though, she recommended that feelings of guilt should not dominate Joan's thinking. A failing heart muscle presented a range of symptoms and signs and many patients delayed seeking help. It was unlikely that Joan's opinion on visiting the doctor was the only factor that played a part.

Roy's narrative

When Alicia visited Roy that afternoon he had already anticipated that she came to tell him off for deciding to leave the programme. Alicia suggested that they start from a different place – his felt needs and what the programme was or was not providing. *You'll judge us on how we think and imagine ways forward, at least I hope that you will*, she told him. She explained that among some patient groups there was a relatively high drop-out rate. She told him that other options existed to address the residual problems of a myocardial infarction, but what was important was what Roy had learned and how he might use that to support himself, irrespective of whether he stayed on or left the programme. Here is part of the conversation that they had.

Alicia: *William's death scared you didn't it. Can you tell me about that?*

Roy: *He just dropped down dead. Nothing they did saved him. All the heroics. The rest of us just stood out in the corridor and gawped.*

Alicia: *It upset my colleague Joanne too. All of you completed the checks before you started exercising as normal. We were desperate to help William.*

Roy: *I don't doubt that you care Alicia, the staff are lovely. But seeing William go, it shook us. Did he have other things wrong with him?*

Alicia: *I can't talk medical details, the confidential things, Roy, but no two patients have exactly the same profile. Risk always attends recovery from an illness. We said at the start, the programme doesn't remove risk entirely.*

Roy: *True. But I started wondering about how confident you could be about judging what stress the heart muscle can handle when you increase the exercise. You're always watching us, checking pulses and blood pressures, but can any of that be precise enough?*

Alicia: *We know, from case histories, a lot about tolerances and what patients can manage. But a key check is the patient working with what they feel they can manage. I'd call it listening to your body and timing out immediately when things seem a bit too much.*

Roy: *Joanne reminded us about that. But I suppose because it's a course and it's only so many weeks long, you start to think that you have to reach a certain level of fitness come what may. I know Joan was always keen that I put the effort in.*

Alicia: *We need some new terminology don't we (she smiled). Course, Programme, it smacks of assessments and performance. Maybe we should call it the tool kit? Let me ask you a different question. Beyond all the things to do and to think about that we teach you, what would seem the absolute best outcome from a programme like ours?*

Roy: *Knowing how to feel safe?*

Alicia: *Feel safe or stay safe?*

Roy: *Feel safe. William showed us that you can't promise us that we'll stay safe.*

Alicia: *OK, so we teach you a lot of things to avoid. We try to help you feel confident taking some carefully graduated exercise. But what would make you feel safe?*

Roy: *I suppose recognising what you didn't spot last time, only much sooner. I suppose it would be knowing that you could take information to your doctor knowing that they would respect what you had noticed and then order the necessary tests. When I collapsed it scared us both.*

Alicia: *So if we could help you find a way to judge tiredness, what you felt before but didn't act on quickly, that would help you?*

Roy: *Yes, certainly.*

Alicia: *Is that as important as lifestyle change, you know, eating the better diet and walking regularly?*

Roy: *Yes, maybe it is. The exercise stuff and the diet stuff, that depends on whether you stick to the regimen. You know that we don't, not all the time! (He laughs.)*

Alicia: *But if we helped you more with reading your health, perhaps by keeping a diary and noting changes over time so that you could see patterns emerging?*

Roy: *Yes.*

Alicia: *People don't keep diaries for very long do they?*

Roy: *They do if they're frightened. They do if they want someone like Joan to understand how they feel. She wants to know that I'm being honest and trusting her to do the helpful thing.*

Alicia: *And if we showed you how to add a few measurements into the diary entries, so that you could show a doctor those changes over time?*

Roy: *Yes, doctors want measurements don't they.*

Alicia:	*If I said, come to the programme days and do the relaxation and the diet bits, and then walk with me rather than exercise, while we talked about some ideas on monitoring tiredness, could you try that?*
Roy:	*You mean that? You'd let me skip the exercise bits?*
Alicia:	*You'd be walking with me while I talk about some possible plans for feeling safe later. If you couldn't talk and walk at the same time, we would know it was time to ease back again. I'm not talking power walking!* (She laughed.)
Roy:	*Did Joan put you up to this?*
Alicia:	*It was something that Joan said, yes. But I've been talking with her about her feelings of guilt, that she didn't stop your heart attack happening.*
Roy:	*She gets some crazy ideas sometimes.*
Alicia:	*If we designed a diary, would you let her read it and perhaps put things in herself, so that you could reflect on what she noticed too?*
Roy:	(smiles) *Why not.*

Activity 6.6   Critical thinking

Look at the dialogue between Alicia and Roy above and jot down what you think Roy's narrative was really about. How did he 'read' the death of his friend? What do you think Alicia's narrative is really about in this extract of dialogue?

An outline answer is provided at the end of the chapter.

Making a plan

After her meeting with Roy, Alicia telephoned his wife. Alicia wanted to assure Joan that what she had asked for had not been forgotten. Alicia wanted to introduce some of the ideas that she had explored with her husband. As Joan was Roy's chief support it seemed important to engage Joan in any plans too. If Roy came to the cardiac rehabilitation days as usual he would continue to derive the benefits of the teaching on diet and stress reduction. Joan was invited to that too. But, instead of completing the exercises, Roy would take a gentler walk with Alicia and make some plans on how they could better monitor for signs or symptoms of recurring heart problems in the future.

Joan sounded relieved. Roy was on his way home and she would talk with him about it that evening. Alicia wondered whether Joan had immediately grasped the subtle shift in programme emphasis that she was now asking Roy to help her explore. As well as gathering things to know about heart disease and lifestyle, to improve exercise tolerance, a future programme might include more help with ways to think about sur-viving a heart attack. It would attend to something that seemed of greater importance to Roy, i.e., how to feel safe. Of course, it would help Joan to feel that progress was being made on weight reduction and diet, but, for Roy, feeling safe preceded that. When they next met, Alicia planned to discuss the diary idea more with Joan. If it worked especially well and Roy increased markedly in his confidence, perhaps Alicia would invite him back to talk to the rehabilitation team about his insights on judging fatigue.

Person-centred care insights

I wonder what you made of Alicia's reasoning in this case study? It's worth tracing some of the insights that she came to while thinking about the support of Roy and his wife Joan. Here they are in summary.

- Alicia started by feeling imperfectly equipped to supply excellent care to Roy and his wife. The fact that the evidence was contradictory left her feeling disappointed. She had, however, forgotten research that related more closely to patient perceptions, the experience and reading of symptoms, and that which sustained a sense of hope.
- Mindful of the evidence deficits, Alicia and her colleagues had already planned some research. This remained important to her as it was about understanding patients and their starting points, but the more that she talked with Roy and his wife Joan the less central that research plan now seemed.
- What did seem of central importance were patient conceptions of risk and relative safety. Both Roy and Joan accepted that risk could not be entirely eliminated. Feeling a little more safe was important though. If ways were found to monitor signs and symptoms better, especially fatigue, then patient and spouse could work to better effect with healthcare professionals.
- Alicia was surprised that Roy seemed to think of the rehabilitation programme in terms such as targets and standards. She was also surprised that Joan conceived of it as treatment. That was not something emphasised by staff. The programme needed to offer patients more emphasis on new ways to think.

Alicia's approach to the case-study circumstances of Roy and Joan are (I think) impres-sive, but let's pause to consider exactly why that is.

Thinking in innovative ways

First, in Chapter 2 I emphasised that in pragmatic person-centred care much of the innovation and the development of new care came from within the care team. It wasn't the case that they simply received a prescription for how care should look, i.e., that recommended by theorists. Person-centred care arose from the imagination of the practitioners themselves. They weren't hide-bound by research to determine how to proceed. For sure, change in a cardiac rehabilitation programme would have to be consulted upon, but the start work begins with an inquisitive attitude and Alicia is well-supplied with inquisitiveness.

Being ready to research

Notice how Alicia and her colleagues were already planning research to better understand patient psychology and their success or otherwise in rehabilitation. This is what might be called problem conception; it is about understanding the extent and the dimensions of a problem. It speculates that a mind-set of the patient, their way of conceiving of the heart in the first place, was linked in some way to whether they were fatalistic about their illness and less confident to use the rehabilitation facilities offered. I wonder whether you too ever conceived of the heart in battery and inevitable failure terms? What is striking, though, is the use of analogy. Patients, Alicia realised, thought of their bodies in terms of analogies. This seems entirely plausible to me.

Being prepared to change

The next way in which Alicia's thinking seems entirely person-centred and impressive relates to what we might call 'think again' mentality. She is willing to reconceive of situations in ways that could improve the service on offer. Alicia isn't without conviction about good care, but she starts with an admission that research evidence is not as perfect as she hoped it would be. But that still leaves opportunities not only to research further, but to explore bespoke adjustments within the programme itself. It would be difficult to persuade Roy to return to the cardiac exercises given the death of his friend William. Statistics on the incidence of cardiac deaths in rehabilitation might not be adequately persuasive. In any case, Roy's primary need at that moment is not exercise per se, it is help with managing fear. Alicia is artful, because while it will take some of her own precious time to work with Roy on the programme days, this remains a sound investment. What she assists Roy with might become a new tool within the programme for other patients. Alicia thinks again and she imagines possibilities. She is operating within the scope of her facilities and both solving problems with Roy but also building possibilities for better service in the future.

Supporting multiple clients

Another way in which Alicia's work impresses relates to her understanding of the care relationship required. It's not the case that nurses care for Roy and then Joan cares for Roy, it is that nurses have to imagine how they can facilitate mutual care within the couple. Whether or not Roy sustains a healthier lifestyle will depend in large degree on his relationship with Joan. She has to be assisted to overcome her feelings of guilt and then acute anxiety, and both need to rebuild a bond of trust. Alicia turns this imaginatively into action by talking to Joan quickly after consulting with Roy on his problem. I think it's possible to imagine the relief, the reassurance, that a prompt telephone call provides. It's also possible to imagine the support that Roy may have felt in realising that Alicia understands quite a lot about his wife's feelings about the heart attack.

Chapter summary

If you read Chapter 5 immediately prior to this one then you will have already been cued in to some debates about rehabilitation courses. Nonetheless, the notion of completing programmes is an essential idea within healthcare, that which delivers health benefits in an effective, efficient and mutually beneficial way. The notion of a programme appeals to the service-minded practitioner on a number of levels. First, it offers an assured product, the component parts are clearly mapped. Second, the programme reminds the patient of the merit of collective action, dealing with problems that they have in common and finding encouragement there. At first sight, however, work within such a programme, as a coordinator for instance, seems to afford much less scope to deliver person-centred care adequately. To use an analogy, it might feel like delivering a set course menu at a restaurant. In this chapter, however, the case is made that there is indeed scope to individualise care within rehabilitation programmes and that patients need not feel lost or ignored within the system that supports them.

- It is important to understand the purposes of rehabilitation. Rehabilitation work is not only directed towards securing and retaining the benefits of recent treatment, but it is also directed at helping patients to cope and to adapt their lifestyle. It is in this psychological area of care that there is particular scope to deliver pragmatic person-centred care.
- Nurses delivering person-centred rehabilitation care are likely to have to move seamlessly back and forth between evidence and patient narratives in order to fashion care suggestions that seem both relevant (patient perception) and clinically sound. The extent to which evidence can help drive person-centred care depends in significant part on the extent to which research has centred on patient experiences and perceived needs. In the relative absence of such evidence, the nurse might have to rely much more heavily on understanding the narratives that the patients and relatives provide.
- It is not the case that the nurse need focus either on the patient as person or on the system that delivers care to a group of patients. It is possible for a nurse (such as Alicia) to discover new thinking benefits that meet both requirements. That which is discovered in consultation with one patient might usefully fuel ideas for the adjustment of a service.

Activities: Brief outline answers

Activity 6.1   Reflecting (p104)

Much of my rehabilitation work centred on altered body image care as I worked with patients dealing with cancer and those recovering from trauma. So the recurring purpose of my work centred again and again on helping patients take back control and improve their resilience. I sometimes shared a speaking platform with representatives of a charity called Changing Faces (**www.changingfaces.org.uk**). Their work also centred on empowering patients to take charge of their new circumstances. Their message was, don't expect others to manage the world around you so that you don't get hurt or feel embarrassed. Decide instead on how you will remodel that world yourself. You are the expert. It was an inspirational message.

Activity 6.2   Reflecting (p105)

It's surprisingly difficult to remember a time when you didn't know more about human anatomy and physiology isn't it. But the exercise is important. Patients don't have our knowledge of the internal body and their conceptions of organs might in some instances be rudimentary. Consider how the heart is conceived of colloquially. People engaged in sports and exercise develop much more sophisticated ideas about the heart, particularly that related to exercise tolerance. They learn about exercise and the endorphin effect on the brain.

Activity 6.3   Critical thinking (p107)

Here are some problems that I noted.

1.   retaining as healthy a heart as possible given the location of the infarction (different patients require different medication dependent upon the location of the blockage).

2.   learning to rethink risk.

3.   learning to re-evaluate the history of the event together (Joan and Roy may have quite different narratives about it).

4.   managing lifestyle habits (dietary, level of activity, etc.).

5.   deliberating on a return to work (thankfully Roy is not engaged in heavy lifting as he drives a forklift truck).

Because Joan and Roy have different narratives about the event it is possible that the heart attack can divide them. Blame and bitterness could affect their subsequent ability to tackle the challenges of the illness. So it is vital that the nurse listens to and understands narratives as well as what evidence might have to offer.

Activity 6.4   Speculating (pp108–9)

The obvious deduction here is that the unclear research evidence on mortality and morbidity post-myocardial infarction can be used to reinforce the patients' instinctive approach to rehabilitation. The fatalistic patient might say, *see, the programmes don't work*, the optimistic patient might observe, *yes! This is worth doing*. It's unwise to misrepresent evidence. If the evidence is ambiguous then that has to be acknowledged. It's then important to explain (simply) why researchers might reach different conclusions and to then weigh up, on balance, the merits of different possible decisions. The decision remains that of the patient, but they usually appreciate hearing the nurse's own rehearsal of the arguments for and against different courses of action.

Activity 6.5   Critical thinking (p111)

I was struck by how symbiotic the two were, that is, that one fuelled the other and that, in some regards, they were mutually dependent on each other. I wouldn't suggest that one was more important than the other. Alicia is 'rescued' by what she remembers from her recent research reading, because it suggests a new way to focus on the problem and on what Roy might need most of all. It absolves her of the need to simply debate with him the merits and demerits of rehabilitation programmes. Research evidence has enabled her to focus quickly on the personal experience of his problem.

Activity 6.6   Critical thinking (p114)

Roy's narrative is certainly about fear isn't it, fear of another heart attack and death resulting from that. But I didn't think that it was a panic fear. He is able to reason that risk is ever-present. In the interim, he reads William's death as a warning not to continue with the exercise programme now. But whether he thinks it's better to wait and build up on exercise later is not clear. Roy might not abstractly think of this in problem terms (he is too close to it), but once Alicia starts to explore ideas with him he is responsive to problem solving as a way forward. Learn what I fear and then tackle that.

Alicia's narrative isn't (I think) pre-formulated. It's explorative and conjectural. She is trying out ideas to see how they might fit. Fit in this instance means:

- helping Roy cope with his experiences;
- reassuring Joan that Alicia will help Roy;
- and re-examining what within the programme isn't entirely right for Roy, now, given the death of his friend William.

The way that Alicia talks is called reflection in action; thinking aloud and speculating. It requires some confidence for the nurse to do this in front of the patient.

Further reading

Corrigan, P (2016) *Principles and Practice of Psychiatric Rehabilitation: An Empirical Approach*, 2nd edition. New York: Guilford Press.

Mental health rehabilitation works intimately with the patient's conception of self and of circumstance, so I recommend this book to you. Look at, for example, Chapter 2, which explores the notion of stigma and how that limits rehabilitation. Chapter 6 on differences between illness and wellness (what I would call wellbeing) is also instructive.

Levine, P (2018) *Stronger After Stroke: Your Road Map to Recovery*, 3rd edition. New York: Springer Publishing.

I think it's a good idea to read at least one book on rehabilitation directed to patients. This book deals with the after-effects of a devastating health event and it addresses lifestyle issues similar to those encountered by heart attack patients.

Southwick, S and Charnet, D (2013) *Resilience: The Science of Mastering Life's Greatest Challenges*, 2nd edition. Cambridge: Cambridge University Press.

One of the purposes of rehabilitation is to promote resilience among patients so this is a rather interesting book. The text isn't entirely focussed on health events, but the case examples all remain relevant. What is it within some people's characters, their ways of thinking, that enable them to then cope well with astonishing psychological challenges?

Useful websites

www.bhf.org.uk/heart-health/living-with-a-heart…/cardiac-rehabilitation

British Heart Foundation: cardiac rehabilitation. This link takes you to a simple explanatory video clip on what is involved in joining a cardiac rehabilitation programme. In many regards it is similar to the one co-ordinated by Alicia. As you view it, consider to what extent it anticipates patient concerns. How clearly does it describe the purpose of rehabilitation?

www.bmj.com/content/351/bmj.h5000

British Medical Journal: What it's like to receive cardiac rehabilitation. This link takes you to a podcast interview with a patient who has completed a cardiac rehabilitation programme. I was struck by how much like Roy he sounded. Narratives may change according to context and this patient tells his story retrospectively to a researcher for a medical journal. The narrative shared with a clinician in the midst of events might be different.

Chapter 7 Helping patients to build and sustain self-care motivation

NMC Standards of Proficiency for Registered Nurses

This chapter will address the following platforms and proficiencies:

Platform 1: Being an accountable professional

At the point of registration, the registered nurse will be able to:

1.9 understand the need to base all decisions regarding care and interventions on people's needs and preferences, recognising and understanding any personal and external factors that may unduly influence your decisions.

1.12 demonstrate the skills and abilities required to support people at all stages of life who are emotionally or physically vulnerable.

1.18 demonstrate the knowledge and confidence to contribute effectively and pro-actively in an interdisciplinary team.

Platform 4: Providing and evaluating care

At the point of registration, the registered nurse will be able to:

4.1 demonstrate and apply an understanding of what is important to people and how to use this knowledge to ensure their needs for safety, dignity, privacy, comfort and sleep can be met, acting as a role model for others in providing evidence based person-centred care.

Chapter aims

After reading this chapter, you will be able to:

- critically examine the ways in which the nurse might work with a patient and others to personalise the support of a patient with a mental illness;
- demonstrate further awareness regarding the need for clinicians to revisit previous care interventions and to think again, building on what you learned in Chapter 2.

Introduction

The case study chapters of this book have explored care at different stages of the professional relationship and I have now moved beyond rehabilitation and into the realms of
self-care and health maintenance. Here, too, it is possible to make care personal, working
closely with the patient's circumstances. In this chapter I would like you to pay particular
attention to the way that Gillian draws on different sources of information, learning lessons from the past and adjusting care with Ted for the future (Chapter 2). This case study
is closely associated with motivating a patient, something that recurs as a challenge in
person-centred care. To succeed, patients must want to be our partners and want to sustain their own contribution over time. To that end, nurses have to consider how best to
enthuse patients, finding common purpose in the care shared. Without an understanding of human motivation it is very hard to secure the benefits of care to date.

Mind (2018) observes that one in six people in England will suffer mental health problems, such as depression or anxiety, within their lifetime. Depression is the leading
cause of disability worldwide (Pols et al., 2017), with 615 million people suffering from
this condition (Counselling Directory, 2018). NICE (2009) observes that adult depression has a high relapse rate with patients suffering repeat bouts of depression during
the course of their lifetime.

Depression may arise in association with clear co-morbidities (such as diabetes mellitus or coronary artery disease) or it may arise in ambiguous circumstances. NICE
guidelines (2009) make it clear that, while a stepped approach to management is
preferred (medication reserved for more severe cases), successful treatments may be
highly dependent on the patient's personal circumstances. What works well for one
patient might not succeed with another. Treatment might focus upon:

- adjustments to the environment (for example, light therapy to counter seasonally
  affective disorder) (Kragh et al., 2017);
- chemical adjustments within the brain secured by antidepressants (Anderson and
  Tapesh, 2013) or Electroconvulsive Therapy (ECT) (Leaver et al., 2018);
- learning new coping behaviours (Cognitive Behavioural Therapy) (Conklin and
  Strunk, 2015);
- understanding and countering negative emotions (Counselling for Depression
  (CfD)) (Goldman et al., 2016);
- or upon more explorative measures such as vagal stimulation (Feldman et al.,
  2013) and acupuncture (Hopton et al., 2014).

That depression admits of a range of possible treatments, often used in combination,
and that NICE (2009) acknowledges that significant further research is needed, all signal that sustaining patient motivation and keeping them well represents a significant
challenge for nurses.

Nurses need to understand what motivates a patient to sustain healthy behaviours, i.e.,
those behaviours that minimise the risk of relapse. In depression this is difficult. One of the

cardinal symptoms of depression is that patients lose hope, feeling that they have limited energy. Without an exploration of motivation with the patient it is much more difficult for the nurse to recommend best treatment. Depression is a condition characterised by:

- depressed mood;
- lost interest/pleasure in activities;
- low energy levels;
- feelings of low self-worth or guilt;
- negativity or feelings of helplessness;
- disturbed sleep and/or appetite.

(Sanders and Hill, 2014)

Therefore, working with motivation is a key concern for the nurse. Recourse to antidepressant medication is rarely the complete solution. The Royal College of Psychiatrists observe that only 50–65 per cent of patients respond to medication, that the drug needs to be taken regularly on seven consecutive days to start demonstrating an effect, and that disciplined self-medication needs to continue for six months if a relapse is to be avoided (Royal College of Psychiatrists, 2009).

Activity 7.1   Reflecting

Pause to consider to what extent you have considered motivation when you have been helping patients. Did you ascertain what seemed to sustain patient motivation and did you then use that to adjust how you worked with them?

An outline answer is provided at the end of the chapter.

Motivation

Much of the research and theory associated with human motivation has been conducted within the occupational rather than the healthcare setting. Occupational psychologists are interested in what sustains a highly motivated workforce.

For the purpose of this chapter two theories are summarised and both can be applied to healthcare contexts (see Figure 7.1).

The first theory was offered by Herzberg (Herzberg, 1966; Alshmemri et al., 2017). Herzberg (1966) argued that we might best understand human motivation in terms of that which rewarded the sense of self, person and achievement, and he called these motivational factors. So, for example, in healthcare, a depressed patient might feel motivated if they could manage without antidepressant medication (the goal). In Herzberg's (1966) Two Factor Theory such intrinsic rewards (that which makes me feel individual and good about myself) are balanced against extrinsic constraints,

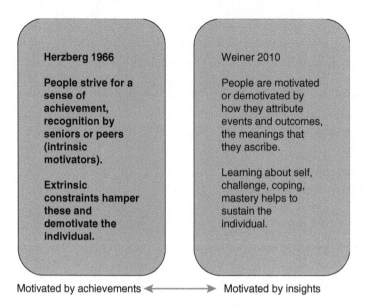

Figure 7.1 boxes:

Herzberg 1966

People strive for a sense of achievement, recognition by seniors or peers (intrinsic motivators).

Extrinsic constraints hamper these and demotivate the individual.

Weiner 2010

People are motivated or demotivated by how they attribute events and outcomes, the meanings that they ascribe.

Learning about self, challenge, coping, mastery helps to sustain the individual.

Motivated by achievements ←————→ Motivated by insights

Figure 7.1 Two theories of motivation

that which restrains the individual from achieving their ideal state. In depression, constraints might include disruption to sleep for example, precisely because this leaves patients tired during the day and less able to cope with their negative thoughts.

Activity 7.2   Critical thinking

Hertzberg's (1966) Two Factor Theory of motivation might have important implications for the work of the nurse. It might, for example, cast the nurse as someone who helps patients look at the constraints in their life in a new light. It might mean that the nurse works to help the patient clarify what they hope to achieve a step at a time. What do you think the positive and the limiting effects of Herzberg's reasoning might be if you tried to understand a patient's motivation using this theory?

An outline answer is provided at the end of the chapter.

The second and more complex theory of motivation shared here comes from Weiner (2010). Weiner is less convinced that people are simply motivated by a reward. He argues that human beings habitually attribute meanings to their behaviour and, through this, they develop a richer sense of who they are. The more the person understands their self the more motivated and reaffirmed they feel. In this theory he argues that we attribute meanings to events and to our behaviour. So, for example, to suffer depression might be explained in terms of predisposing factors, that which made us more prone to the illness. So, to illustrate, a patient might observe that they always struggle to relate to other people and that this isolates them. Understanding their self then provides a key for improvement. Learning about self becomes motivating as we start to reconceive of ourselves as people capable of adapting.

Whether or not you agree with Weiner probably depends on the extent to which you think human beings are self-analytical. If you think that we constantly evaluate and re-evaluate our actions, then you might be more inclined to find Weiner's theory appealing. What is important about his theory, however, is not the particular attributions that we use to explain what is happening to us and how well we are doing, it is what characterises those attributions. We can explain this using three questions.

1. How stable is that attribution? (Do I explain things the same way all of the time? If I do, we might question whether this seems helpful.)

2. How much control do people have in these matters? (It is important to forgive the self if no control could humanly be exercised.)

3. How much control did I exercise about these events and what does that say about me? (We carry responsibility for our responses to some situations that arise.)

The important observation relating to Weiner's attribution theory is that it offers a potential profile of successful coping. The person who redefines events and their responses in more positive ways is much more likely to go on succeeding and they may be less susceptible to problems in the future. Respecting oneself and one's efforts is critical to endeavour. In a world where there is greater access to social media and therefore comparison of our social performance, i.e., how well we do and how much we are liked, this might be extremely important.

Activity 7.3   Critical thinking

Pause now to contemplate Weiner's theory of motivation. What implications might it have for explaining why some depressed patients might struggle to sustain health? What might this theory offer with regard to helping the patient understand their emotions, i.e., that which can lock them inside an illness and potentially pose significant demands on their family?

An outline answer is provided at the end of the chapter.

Depression

Salmon (2017), reporting OECD (Organisation for Economic Cooperation and Development) statistics, observes that the UK ranks joint seventh in the world for the incidence of depression. While there are growing numbers of statistics relating to the high incidence of the problem, explanations of how depression arises and what distinguishes it from other conditions are much less clear. Patients, for example, frequently report a mix of symptoms relating to depression and anxiety. NICE (2009) argues that depression can be diagnosed when symptoms have been present for at least two weeks and affect the individual most days during that period. NICE observes, however, that a full patient history is needed, setting the arrival of problems in a life context.

What is clearer is that depression represents a significant burden on relatives (Skundberg-Kletthagen et al., 2014). The persistent nature of depression symptoms and periodic crises in patients means that relatives suffer a loss of control over their own lives. Relatives reported living on the patient's terms. Depression increased the chances that the relationship between the patient and their family became ambivalent. Relatives became suspicious of the patient's illness and pessimistic as to whether it could improve. Relatives struggled to fulfil their own social roles as well as to act as a carer.

Frank et al. (2007) described the experience of depression as reported within focus-group discussions. While group discussions might help with a variety of things, it was often feelings of irritability with self (my coping) that were often relieved. Patients frequently judged themselves and their response to depression and irritability increased their despair. In a rare study exploring patient perceptions of why depression arose and why it persisted, Kelly et al. (2011) proposed that strained interpersonal relationships featured in the experience of illness. Patients who became lonely, who felt alienated from others and isolated, struggled more to deal with their negative emotions. It was debatable whether the strained social relationships occasioned depression or whether they resulted from it (a chicken and egg conundrum), but this study does seem to confirm that the way we attribute meanings to our way of living is important in shaping the experience of illness over time.

Kelly et al. (2011) suggest that two processes may be underway within depression.

1. First, uncomfortable experiences and emotions are internalised, so that patients feel that the illness is their fault. They may feel sorry for themselves and this can prove especially wearing for relatives.

2. The second process, though, exacerbates the problem, with patients behaving aggressively towards those who try to help them. The patient is alarmed at their own unattractive negative emotions, i.e., that which they define as undignified, and then they become anxious about the best means to cope. Patient narratives are therefore important to finding the better therapeutic interventions. Depression is both an illness associated with behaviour (e.g., withdrawal) and with perception (the patient's self-judgement).

Eliciting narratives from patients can be difficult, especially if they presume that their thoughts and feelings are unattractive or shameful in some way. However, the nurse has a greater chance of success where he or she does the following.

- Highlights that doubts feature strongly as part of the illness. It is therefore legitimate for the patient to express concerns about how the problems have been coped with.

- Indicates that he or she understands that illnesses are complex and change over time. It is only by mapping how they change, through the patient's thoughts and feelings, that healthcare professionals can adequately respect and help the patient.

Activity 7.4   Reflecting

Doblyte and Jimenez-Mejias (2017), in their review of research, explain that some patients see help-seeking as a threat to their personal integrity and fear seeming highly dependent on others.

In your experience, do you think that you are harder to help if you feel angry with your efforts to achieve a desired outcome? What, within your experience of coping and help-receiving, might seem important when you consider ways to help depressed patients in a person-centred way?

As this activity is based on your own reflection, no sample answer is provided at the end of the chapter.

Case study: Ted

Last January Ted reached the age of 70. A retired aeronautical engineer, he approached his seventh decade with some trepidation. Six years ago he had lost his wife Grace to lung cancer. As Ted saw it, they were robbed of a retirement together and of the travels that they had put off because of work. Grace had been in and out of hospital for 14 months receiving palliative treatment. For that period Ted had been his wife's chief carer. Ted didn't remember getting much sleep and sometimes that meant he became irritable with his wife even though he understood just how ill she was.

A few months after Grace's death, Ted had visited his GP to discuss how low he felt. Ted assumed that this was all to do with grief, but wondered just how long the feelings of despair were meant to continue. His friends were worried that he had not *chirped up* again. One friend had suggested bereavement counselling but Ted had insisted that he and his wife hadn't been youngsters. Death was part of life and one had to adapt. Still, adaptation seemed to take a long time. Ted's GP told him that the distinctions between mourning, grief and depression were necessarily vague, but that what he had described was sufficiently concerning that it might be a good idea to complete a six-month course of an antidepressant Fluoxetine (Prozac) to help him complete his recovery from the loss of his wife. Ted learned that the drug should help improve his mood. For it to work

(Continued)

(Continued)

though, he would need to take his medication daily and visit the surgery monthly so that its effect could be monitored.

The doctor explained that Ted also needed to deal with the underlying causes of his low mood. It was important to talk about the loss of his wife and any other negative feelings. To that end, the doctor recommended a course of Cognitive Behavioural Therapy (CBT). Medication was only one weapon in the armoury used to counter depression.

Ted coped reasonably well with his medication and completed the six-month course with relatively few missed tablet days. At the end of his course of medication, however, Ted was anxious to wean himself off his drugs and to find better ways to cope. Despite the doctor's advice he hadn't taken up offers of a talking therapy. Now, aged 70, staring bleakly into the future, Ted felt sure that his illness was back. Ted had given up playing golf (something that both Grace and he had enjoyed) and now he stayed up late into the night listening to the news. He admitted that the news stories were on loops in his head and went around and around but he felt he couldn't let go of them. At the time of his illness there were a lot of debates about the economy and Ted had a gloomy feeling that the country was heading towards ruin. Spending a great deal of time worrying about politics, Ted suffered a fitful sleep. He found it hard to drag himself out of the bed in the morning and wondered what there was left to get up for. When you were 70, well, the decades ahead, if you had them at all, were decades of inevitable decline.

Now, at last, after some 'bullying' by an old friend of his from the golf club, Ted has been persuaded to join a book club. His friend (Michael) insisted that reading and discussing novels *stopped you maudling*. But Ted simply goes through the motion of discussing books and a nurse (Gillian) who also attends the book club noticed his emotional flatness. Ted rarely smiled. Ted struggled to express passion or pleasure about what the novels cover and yet they were indeed provocative reads. Gillian, who works with a mental health self-help group, was worried that Ted might slip back into acute depression. She noted that he talked about few friends save for Michael and had comparatively little social intercourse save for the book club meetings once a fortnight.

Activity 7.5   Speculating

Jot down what you think Ted's problems are and the ways in which these are very personal. Do you think that the help he has received so far has been as comprehensive as it should have been? Why might it be more difficult to personalise the care for a patient such as Ted?

An outline answer is provided at the end of the chapter.

Attending to the needs and the concerns of the patient

Gillian wasn't surprised that Ted was starting to run into difficulties again. Patients with depression rather easily slipped beneath the radar of the caring services and, as a result, they tended to return to acute care facilities again and again. From what Ted had summarised, he had received a part-treatment. While his course of Fluoxetine had lifted his mood pro tem, it had not addressed his underlying problems. Goldman et al. (2016) observe that only some 25 per cent of patients secure a coherent and complete treatment package. This was often because the patient accepts some elements of treatment and abandons others. NICE (2009) advocate combination modalities of treatment, often a medication such as Fluoxetine and a talking therapy such as Cognitive Behavioural Therapy. While the medication works physiologically to lift the mood of the patient, the talking therapy operates to help the patient adjust their perceptions of their circumstances.

NICE (2009) guidelines advocate a stepped approach to care with medication reserved for well-established and moderate to severe depression. In step one, interventions advocated are psycho-educational in nature (for example, a self-help group) and include regular monitoring. But the problem with this approach is that a healthcare professional might not define the patient's problem as established depression. In this case study, the well-meaning GP saw the problem as one of grief and hoped that a course of antidepressant medication might help carry the patient through the transition. Recommendation was made that Ted begin a talking therapy as well but this had not been adequately followed up.

The Talking Sense (2018) initiative describes depression as an emotional problem complicated by interpersonal processes. Patients are often self-critical and difficult to assist and they may have actively subverted efforts to help them. When patients are then offered medication by a well-meaning clinician the underlying problems can remain unaddressed. General practitioners as well as other clinicians are aware of the ambiguous success rates of treatments, so it is extremely tempting to offer medication if the patient argues that they would appreciate a pill that *tides them over.*

Anderson and Tapesh (2013) reviewed patient experiences of taking antidepressant medication and observed that the use of such drugs has doubled within the last decade. But using such drugs often created conflicting issues for patients. Some patients hated feeling dependent on the drugs, but others reported some significant relief from the symptoms of depression. However, the way in which the medication was introduced and explained was sometimes key to whether patients coped well with their medication. Some patients became cynical both about drugs and the professionals who recommended them.

One of the problems with commending a stepped approach to care for Ted was that there were conflicting arguments about whether the approach was viable. Pols et al. (2017), reporting on their own study with Danish patients suffering depression, admitted that the results were mixed. One of the problems was that the stepped approach often involved protracted periods of time persevering with a less intrusive form of therapy (at least three months) and that this meant that sometimes a problem might not be adequately addressed for a year or more. Against this, other studies (Van Veer-Tazelaar et al., 2009; Dozeman et al., 2012; Van der Aa et al., 2015) all reported relatively good results. There were three things that were critical to the success of the stepped approach:

1. adequate well-co-ordinated talking therapy resources;
2. a systematic approach to assessment and early stage guidance of the patient (the same case worker, for example);
3. conviction about the merits of talking therapies.

Unfortunately, within the UK, clinicians and advisors are sometimes ambivalent about one or other talking therapy and this means that patients might be sent to a service more associated with staff confidence than what might suit an individual patient best. Gillian was concerned that considerations about the cost of different treatments, the commitment required of patients, and whether outcomes could be measured, might determine whether the treatment was the right fit for the patient. In Gillian's experience, clinicians sometimes forgot what might motivate a patient.

One of the most common talking therapies used to assist patients with depression is Cognitive Behavioural Therapy. In this treatment patients are helped to understand how their way of reasoning creates behaviours that might trap them within a current problem. The therapist then works with the patient through a series of exercises (new behaviours) that can confirm to the patient that they are capable of living differently. Conklin and Strunk (2015) described this approach to patients suffering from depression and emphasised that the 'homework' set between one-to-one therapist meetings was key to the success of the programme. The number of sessions that a patient needed to secure progress might be determined by the extent to which patients engaged with activity homework set between times. Such a talking therapy approach might work for Ted, but it depended rather on whether he would commit to the homework activities and whether he saw sustaining health as something that could be learned and practised in a behavioural way. It was a possibility. Ted was an engineer and the methodical and analytical approach might work.

Against that, however, it also seemed important to Gillian to think about the psychosocial elements of depression as well. Ted had withdrawn from the golf club, something that he and his wife enjoyed. It was important to understand why Ted had given up this source of support, especially when his friend Michael came from that background. Ted didn't have any remaining close friends and, as depression was taxing on others, it seemed a promising idea to re-engage Ted with his golf club where a wider group of people might help to sustain Ted's morale. Nystrom and Nystrom (2007) had emphasised how recurrent depression had the potential to alienate a patient from others and from their self. Others became, in the Nystroms' terms, the reasons why 'patients wanted to live or to die', so it seemed important to understand how Ted viewed the golf club and help-giving before recommendations were made.

Activity 7.6   Critical thinking

Gillian is willing to be responsibly critical of the service afforded to Ted and to try to learn lessons going forward from that. This isn't, however, a matter of inter-professional 'point scoring'. Why do you think it important that she revisits what was missing from Ted's passage of care to date?

An outline answer is provided at the end of the chapter.

Gillian proposed three things to Ted:

1. First, that he join her support group, for which there was no charge. The group engaged in a range of activities designed to start people thinking about the wider world and which enabled them to secure mutual support. Activities included visits to the cinema, book reviewing, nature walks, visits to art galleries and similar.

2. In order to proceed, though, Gillian explained that she would wish to consult with Ted's GP, explaining the services that she could offer. This was a matter of professional etiquette. General practitioners had their own support and talking therapies network that they regularly used and it was important that Ted received a joined-up support and wasn't drawn into a conflict over who looked after the patient. Ted admitted that he had ignored the invitation to start Cognitive Behavioural Therapy. The GP surgery had sent him two letters about that. Gillian said that she wasn't sure which talking therapy might help Ted most; the charity she worked for had access to several. She hoped to explore with Ted what his needs might be. It was necessary to work with what motivated and sustained Ted best.

3. That Ted revisit his GP to describe his failing mood and recommence antidepressant medication. Gillian wasn't prepared to involve Ted in the group work until such time as this matter had been clarified by his GP. Gillian wanted to know that she had colleague support to contribute to his care and then she could operate in a way that worked with any medication that he was prescribed.

Ted agreed to the proposals and, a week later, Gillian visited the GP to discuss how they might work together. The GP was disgruntled that Ted had not simply raised his recurring problem with him so that treatment of different kinds could be recommenced. He thought it may have been valuable to try bereavement counselling even though Ted was some time away from the death of his wife. Gillian assured him that the assessment she had offered was happenchance and through a book club. It had seemed impossible not to attend to Ted's state and she was eager to work with the GP to help Ted now.

Ted recommenced his medication and the GP agreed that Ted would join the support group and access a talking therapy there, provided that he was adequately consulted on proposals made.

Activity 7.7   Speculating

Gillian is setting in train (with the GP) three elements of support. There is a renewed medication designed to help lift Ted's mood. There is a support group to assure Ted that he is not alone in dealing with his problems. There will then be a carefully chosen talking therapy that helps Ted to reason in a new way about his situation. How do you think the combination of three supports might work to enable Ted to feel that his care is appropriately person-centred?

An outline answer is provided at the end of the chapter.

Hearing the patient narrative

The support group that Ted attended offered its own forms of support, but it also afforded the chance for Gillian to talk to Ted on a regular basis. Groups are often beneficial in eliciting patient narratives. First, the patient shares their feelings with fellow sufferers and then, later, the nurse or therapist can pick up on themes that emerged there. She learned about the help that Michael had provided and the important part that the golf club had played in Ted's past life. While Ted's wife Grace had died some years ago, Gillian wanted to understand the narrative of living that Ted had developed since. This was important for three reasons. First, the way that Ted talked about these matters would give a clue as to his emotional state and indicate whether his medication was once again assisting him. Second, hearing Ted's stories of what had happened since Grace had gone, might help characterise how Ted narrated his life (the attributions that he made). For example, did he characterise himself as a struggler, or someone who was condemned to live in a particular way? Third, Gillian wanted to understand what motivated Ted best before exploring with him and his GP which talking therapy might best protect him from future problems.

Three important patient conversations

Reviewing Ted's care a few weeks later, four conversations stood out for Gillian. Three of the conversations were with Ted and the fourth was with his GP. The first memorable conversation with Ted related to his wife Grace. It was suffused with love for his deceased wife but also a growing bitterness that he had not contributed more to their relationship. One passage stood out. Ted said,

I was angry that the cancer took Grace from me, before we could have our holidays together. I was angry that it made me her nurse when she was ill at the end. Then, though, it was awful. I've started to think how fed up I am with myself because, for most of my married life, I let her do the organising. Grace organised me and most of what I did. When I wasn't at work, I did things that Grace had organised for us. The golf club was good, but it was as much for her as it was for me because the ladies section played bridge there as well.

It shocked Ted that he resented his wife and despised himself. He clearly loved her dearly but, subsequent to her death, it had been surprising to realise that he had simply let her make so many decisions. It had just been convenient to accept her plans and in Ted's view that was not *proper partnering*. Now that his wife was gone he couldn't rectify that. Ted felt very angry with himself for being lazy and unimaginative.

The second conversation with Ted related to his friend Michael at the golf club. Michael had consistently and quietly offered his support to Ted, much of which Ted admitted he brushed off as interfering. But Ted was struggling to understand why he resented Michael's offer of help. Here is an excerpt of Ted's narrative about that.

I shouldn't be rude to Michael, I shouldn't. He only means to help me. I know that, but it's always at the wrong time and in the wrong way. It's as if he is a busy body and he won't accept that. He's trying his best but he irritates the hell out of me.

Gillian concluded that there remained some form of interpersonal difficulty for Ted and that Michael might be representative of that. It was possible that it was because Michael represented the golf club, something that linked Ted back to Grace in a painful way. It was possible that the golf club represented a challenge, one where Ted might have to explain his *dark and pessimistic thoughts*.

The third memorable conversation related to reaching the age of 70. Ted's problems were not solely associated with grief. Gillian realised that Ted hadn't decided what you were meant to be like when you reached the seventh decade. Ted didn't have a narrative that explained how you were meant to feel, what you were meant to do. Now that Ted wasn't playing golf any more, how was he meant to fill his day? Ted seemed to assume that, by the seventh decade, your physical health was meant to shut off activities such as golf.

I suppose something will set in. There is arthritis in the family. Sometimes I look at my fingers and wonder why they don't yet ache. I get out of bed and know that one morning soon my back will have gone and I will be on the downward slope. What's the point then? You can only read so many books. Grace was the book reader not me. The odd crime novel maybe, but books alone, Christ!

Ted's seventh decade narrative was one of inevitable and awaited decline. He had no conception of just how physically active some people were in their seventh, eighth and even ninth decade. Gillian found a picture of Prince Phillip driving carriages with a team of horses when he was considerably older than Ted. Rapid physical decline in old age was not inevitable.

A discourse with the GP

The fourth memorable conversation came when she visited Ted's GP to commend a particular talking therapy. She anticipated that the GP would wish her to arrange CBT sessions for Ted or perhaps to consider again bereavement counselling. Gillian, however, wished to propose instead Counselling for Depression (CfD), a form of support that helped the patient to explore what their emotional problems were and to accept and respect themselves for what they did to understand their difficulties (Goldman et al., 2016). Ted's problems may have centred first on the death of his wife but they were bigger than that now. Counselling for Depression sessions didn't proceed ad infinitum. Like CBT, it comprised a course lasting circa 12 weeks and was arranged as weekly one-to-one sessions. Her linked therapist (Jason) had trained specifically in CfD in 2011 and he had already helped two other patients who were referred to him. Counselling for Depression worked for different patients in different ways, but she was prepared to argue the case to the GP. Here is an excerpt from that conversation.

GP: *Ted has seemed a good deal more settled because of your support group Gillian. I'm pleased.*

Gillian: *It works better some weeks than others. Sometimes I find myself rescuing them all because they feel negative on the same day.*

GP: *Nonetheless, Ted values it. His face is more animated when he describes his visits to the group. So we need to discuss talking therapy now. I don't want Ted to miss out again. I let him slip the net last time and we need to ensure that what we do now isn't wasted.*

Gillian: *I agree and I want to make a pitch to you. I want to suggest something that possibly isn't so obvious.*

     I've made some notes about my conversations with Ted over the last few weeks and they suggest several things. First, Ted is still trying to make sense of why he is so miserable. Second, he is quite angry with himself. Ted isn't the methodical person that he thinks he should be. While losing Grace is important in this, it's bigger than that. For example, Ted doesn't know what he wants to be at 70.

GP: *Existential angst.* (He smiles.)

Gillian: *Yes! I mean it practically though. Ted meets miserable emotions every day. But some come up from his memory. He remembers and regrets things about how he thinks that he should have lived with his wife. He then seems to use that against himself. He uses that to hate himself a bit. But he ponders, too, on how you should be as you age.*

GP: *If Ted could understand that, how he behaves, then he could understand why he gets stuck with this.*

Gillian: *I know CBT. But I want to tempt you to another place. CBT is firmly learning and problem solving. The therapist has to work quite briskly to clarify the problem and to then teach how that fuels unhelpful behaviour. That will push Ted along quite fast. There's a risk that he won't do the homework. He already resists pushy help from his friend Michael. I think that we have to suggest something that is more likely to motivate Ted.*

GP: *You feel that CBT wouldn't work?*

Gillian: *I feel that it wouldn't work so well for Ted right now. Ted is still assigning meanings to what he feels and what that involves for how he lives. I suspect that Ted would appreciate help with that work first. Another time, perhaps if his illness comes back, CBT might be right. But for now I'd like to suggest Counselling for Depression. I know someone, an excellent, hard-headed counsellor. We fund the first course of counselling, after that the charity can't provide more. You could keep your CBT facilities for later … if needed.*

GP: *OK, I have a suggestion. We ask Ted to write up reflections afterwards. That way I can learn some more about the counselling. I've never referred anyone to that before.*

Gillian: *That would be due diligence.*

GP: *Yes.* (He smiled.)

Subsequently Gillian proposed counselling support to Ted. She described how Jason worked and recommended an exploratory meeting to see whether Ted could feel comfortable working with the therapist. Therapy could explore how anger could make a problem more difficult to unravel. It might explain how forgiving yourself could help you feel a little more positive. What Ted decided post therapy would remain firmly his business. But it was possible that the therapy could help him to clarify what he wanted to do. The support group would remain; that was always there. In the meantime, using his medication again and exploring how feelings arose and loomed so large could prove a fruitful combination.

Ted agreed to meet with the therapist and added that he should have been ready for it before. *No,* said Gillian, *you are ready for it when you feel ready for it. Life is more than a performance.*

Activity 7.8   Critical thinking

Look back now at the excerpt of dialogue that Gillian shared with the GP. How does she present her case so as to persuade the GP to support the plan she wants to offer Ted?

An outline answer is provided at the end of the chapter.

Person-centred care insights

This case study offers a number of quite powerful insights into person-centred care.

Helping patients amid their illness

The first insight relates to the nature of the illness. Some illnesses are strongly physiologically centred. But an illness such as depression is very perceptual in nature. The way that an individual experiences their emotions, the responses of others and then judges their own efforts to counter problems is influenced by their perceptions. Wherever personal sense-making forms a large part of what counts as illness and what seems workable as treatment, person-centred care becomes that much more important (Sanders and Hill, 2014). Without attending closely to the patient's experiences and their perceptions, healthcare work might be wasted and even prove counterproductive. Clinicians need to listen to the narratives shared by patients, so that the 'felt situation' is understood. You may identify a range of other conditions that mix the need for a physical and an individualised therapy response. For example, cancer patients might both utilise treatments that counter a tumour but also use talking therapies that help them to live with the episode of illness and associated treatment.

Discovering feelings through narratives

I think that the second intensely person-centred-care element of this case study relates to narrative. To understand what a person 'suffers' clinicians have to hear the patient narrative. That narrative offers clues not only about the felt needs of the patient but also what sorts of solutions and comforts might be most welcome to them. In this example, Ted is struggling to understand his emotions, but he is also wrestling with the gut reactions that he has to them and the judgements that he makes upon himself since the loss of his wife. Making sense of these, perhaps forgiving himself for judged shortfalls, might be materially useful in helping Ted to manage his depression. Whatever medication offers in terms of an improved mood, that is best sustained when the patient learns how they can take over from the drug, sustaining self-respect in the weeks or months ahead.

Eliciting narratives is a key skill of the person-centred care nurse. There may be no formulaic way to ensure that narratives are secured, especially when supporting patients with a mental illness, but in my experience each of the following has merit.

- Establishing a respect for the emotions that the patient feels. Misery is not something to be criticised out of hand. However frightening it is for you to think 'what if I became depressed', it is a state that the patient finds themselves in and you need to say that you understand and respect that.
- Sharing the fact that you have doubts too. Depressed patients often forget that doubt and uncertainty are part of the human condition. They may criticise themselves for it as an entirely personal failing. If you admit that you are sometimes unsure how to proceed, then you show that it is human to work things out as you go along.

- Inviting the patient to elaborate on their thoughts by posing open questions, those that don't readily allow a 'yes or no' answer. So, it might be helpful to ask, 'so how have you felt over the last few days?' 'What seems to have changed and what seems to remain the same for you?'

Creating better narratives

You might have noted two other regards in which hearing narratives were important in this case study. The first of these is concerned with the fact that managing depression is largely about creating a new narrative. Ted has to discover a new way to story-tell himself as a 70-year-old. He has to find a new story to tell about being a widower. Another regard in which narrative is important is that narratives determine whether successful treatments can be identified and agreed. Gillian anticipates that the GP might feel much more cautious about CfD. Her own narrative is about patient choice and making a good use of therapy. But without thinking about the other clinician's comfortable narratives, and listening and responding to the same, she is less likely to argue a potentially helpful course of action. You need to attend, to hear, to think and to respond sensitively.

Thinking again about care

A further person-centred care insight that I identified related to the willingness of clinicians to think again, to acknowledge shortfalls and mistakes, and to innovate. This was particularly important in this case because there is not currently the same body of evidence supporting the value of CfD as there is for CBT. NICE (2009) acknowledges that much remains to be learned about the successful management of adult depression, but, in the interim, it's quite possible that clinicians will err on the side of more familiar therapies. For Gillian to make a successful case about this she needed a good knowledge of the evidence available to date and clear convictions about why a particular therapy might benefit a patient at a particular stage of their illness. In this instance, that which commends CfD over CBT is not an ideological commitment to one or other treatment, but the proximity of what it attempts to do with the indicated needs in the patient narrative. Person-centred care is about fit of therapy.

Linking therapy to motivation

I wonder if you spotted that Gillian was using Weiner's (2010) theory of motivation? She believed that Ted was in the midst of still attributing values to his past way of living, his response to his wife's death and the challenges of being 70 years old. Ted was still in his *murky depths of making sense of it all*. It was Gillian's supposition that if Ted was helped to understand his emotions and the anger that seemed to weave that together, he might respect himself more and start to enjoy the realisation of his own insights. The more Ted understood himself and his circumstances, the greater the potential there seemed for him to self-care in the future. Ted was confronting what it meant to be retired alone, to be widowed and to contemplate what ageing might bring in the future. Gillian's discussion with the GP centred upon narrative insights with Ted. The GP was willing to explore a new therapy approach, especially if that could afford new clinical insights as well. But had the dialogue faltered, one of the things that Gillian could have done would have been to explain how individuals might be motivated. An understanding of psychology, from a completely different field of practice, might have utility in healthcare.

Chapter summary

This chapter highlights the importance of understanding motivation as part of supporting a patient suffering from depression. Depressed patients face particular challenges in self-motivating themselves. Person-centred care, then, is closely associated with discovering what might motivate a patient, and to do that the nurse has to elicit a rich narrative of patient experiences and thoughts and project that forward when recommending treatment and support measures.

Person-centred care needs to operate not only when patients are acutely ill, recovering and rehabilitating, but it might also need to come into play when you help to keep patients well. For that to work successfully the nurse must understand the person and how that person is currently trying to live. Living is not a given, it can falter and, especially in depression, patients can start to slip back into problems that seem much harder to escape from. The timely offer of support, the imaginative mixing of care suggestions and the brave liaison work with fellow professionals are part of what feature in excellent person-centred care.

- Remaining well is not necessarily a passive matter. Many patients, especially those who suffer from depression, have to work at self-care. For nurses to work with patients on such matters you need to understand what motivates them. The more you understand motivation the better you can match support suggestions and treatment options to beneficial effect.
- Illness involves experiences and perceptions. The patient experiences symptoms in a personal context and they also evaluate their coping in that setting. For care to work you need to understand the patient's context and the extent to which they have made sense of what is wrong. Attenuating symptoms alone is not an adequate person-centred response.
- A recommended treatment needs to match the patient's state of readiness to use it. Therapies represent tools and wise care relates to choosing the right time to use each tool.
- Improving patient care, however, making it more person-centred, starts with humility. Clinicians and patients sometimes make mistakes and fail to utilise a resource at the time it would be most valuable. There is often a need to think again and to liaise in ways that help the patient to understand why you are inviting them to partner actively with you.

Activities: Brief outline answers

Activity 7.1   Reflecting (p123)

Candidly, I have not always considered patient motivation enough. I have tended to return to motivation when the patient's progress has faltered. I have tended to use motivation insights as a rescue response, especially when I used to help patients to live with disfigurement.

But I now think that understanding motivation is pivotal to demonstrating person-centred care. When you ask a patient what sustains them, what motivates them, you signal very quickly indeed an interest in what matters most to them and what reassures them. Understanding and using motivation theory is part of the person-centred-care counter to trite prescription. Instead of saying that you have illness X and the response here is therapy Y, you acknowledge that therapies are tools for patients. Patients take the pills, patients turn up for the talking therapy sessions and they labour emotionally by completing activities there. Patients attend and contribute to support groups. If the patients do so much of the work then you need to consider what sustains them in that.

Activity 7.2   Critical thinking (p124)

One of the positives of Herzberg's (1966) theory of motivation is that it highlights a form of reasoning that patients are likely to find relatively easy to understand. We make a lot of life decisions based on effort and reward. It's heroic to overcome the odds: I'll stick at this diet and then have one slap-up meal when I have reached my target weight. We are accustomed to identifying rewards to sustain our efforts. One of the problems, though, is that many patients' circumstances are a little more complex than that. Someone suffering from a chronic illness, such as depression, has to identify repeated rewards for themselves, and the fact that these aren't sustainable, that they seem less enjoyable or fulfilling, limits the utility of this theory. There are many conditions where patients spend more time making sense of their illness, something that cannot so easily be reduced to factors that motivate and those that constrain.

Activity 7.3   Critical thinking (p125)

One of the problems for depressed patients is that they think in the midst of their illness. The very process of reasoning is affected by their emotional state, the anxiety and the low expectation of hope that may operate there. Patients are still attributing meanings to what is happening and how they are responding. Until they can name the emotional and the reasoning problems, it is much harder for the patient to counteract the negatives encountered. So Weiner's theory is quite compelling in these circumstances. It may be possible to understand how and why we attribute things to what has happened or what we have done. If we can understand why we feel we are a failure, if we understand why we fear that people will not like us, we can start to unravel how those sets of perceptions and beliefs produce the mental state we experience. One of the merits of using antidepressant medication in combination with a talking therapy is because the drug can help lift a mood and give space for a new form of reasoning to operate for the patient. That reasoning in some therapies centres strongly on reviewing emotions and forgiving ourselves for our imperfections.

Activity 7.5   Speculating (p128)

Even before you consider his narrative, Ted seems to have some likely problems. First, there is a problem relating to grief. Ted feels robbed of his wife and the retirement time he anticipated with her. But Ted also seems to have lost volition to continue with activities from the past. His friend Michael has to pursue him to commit to something. Ted cautiously takes his medication, but he hasn't availed himself of a talking therapy in harness with that treatment. There is a risk that a symptom (low mood) might be temporarily alleviated but that the underlying processes that have fuelled it won't have been addressed. Perhaps, then, the chief problem that Ted faces is that he is unsure what he is doing to get better. He follows GP advice as regards the use of a drug, but he hasn't understood why a talking therapy sustains what that medication might afford in the short term.

Activity 7.6   Critical thinking (p131)

Realistically, whatever the GP advised Ted about adjuvant talking therapy, no matter how he was reminded of that, the fact is that he completed a course of medication alone and this was less likely to help him sustain his wellbeing longer term. Gillian needed to revisit that deficit with Ted and the GP in order to give a clearer purpose to the support next recommended. Different therapies work to different ends. For example, medication operates to change mood within the patient. A support group operates to reassure the patient when other lay support might not be available or sustainable. A talking therapy operates to help the patient reason in a new way so that coping can be improved. But, for any combination of support to succeed in the future, Ted needs to appreciate why a part response in the past was less successful.

Activity 7.7   Speculating (p132)

I would suggest that the fact that Gillian has negotiated a combination of support with him will help Ted to feel that care is tailor-made. Care services are not infinite but, in this instance, the GP is working with a charity to enable a patient to receive something that might work well. Ted knows that he is difficult to help and he appreciates that Michael has tried to support him. So attending a group and working with a therapist might help him to understand how irritability gets in the way of progress. It is just this sort of attention to detail that suggests to a patient that you have due concern for their experiences and problems.

Activity 7.8   Critical thinking (p135)

We don't know what the GP knows or thinks about CfD. Gillian didn't either, but she begins cautiously, using her experience of other medical responses to counselling approaches. It was Gillian's experience that counselling was seen by medical colleagues as less effective, that it was inherently less focussed and that it might continue for a long time to little clinical benefit. So Gillian started with a clear strategy. She hopes to establish her collaborative interest in Ted with the GP and to demonstrate a due critical humility about her own work. Note how she observes that the group work isn't invariably successful every day. She guesses that the GP might already feel judged by the failure of the past care approach.

Her strategy is to demonstrate her understanding of Ted and his needs. Notice how she refers to her notes and provides examples of what sorts of problems Ted has. It is much harder for a busy GP to have got to the bottom of this given available consultation time. Once she has established an interest in patient need and readiness to use a talking therapy, Gillian can move towards her preferred recommendation. Counselling for Depression is not an ideological choice. It is not CfD versus CBT. It's a consultation on the right tool for the job. By starting with patient need Gillian sidesteps any debate about rights to prescribe. The GP and the nurse commend the next step forward together, and the GP is reassured of the merits of this course by her report of the professionalism of Jason the counsellor and by the fact that the intervention will be evaluated later.

Further reading

Lewis, G (2016) *Sunbathing in the Rain: A Cheerful Book About Depression.* London: Harper Perennial.

It is possible to write about an illness with both wit and insight. Geraldine Lewis manages that and then some. As depression is potentially a lifelong illness with recurrence of problems over time, a memoire is well-suited to offering patient insights.

Sanders, P and Hill, A (2014) *Counseling for Depression: A Person-Centred and Experiential Approach to Practice.* London: SAGE.

Given the incidence of depression as an illness in society it seems valuable for all nurses to understand how this affects patients and what therapists try to do to alleviate suffering. One of the problems that can attend depression is the public perception that it is difficult or impossible to treat. The more that nurses convey optimism that one or other, or perhaps a combination, of therapies can assist, the more they may help patients to address their problems.

Useful websites

www.ted.com/.../andrew_solomon_depression_the_secret_w...

Andrew Solomon (2013) *Depression: The Secret We Share.* TED Ideas Worth Spreading. I recommend this 30-minute video talk by Andrew Solomon to you. It shows how depression is more than grief and how it can profoundly shape how people interpret their lives. Solomon observes that people with depression believe that happiness is a veil that has been removed. They believe that they live with the truth and that the truth is that we will all die and that there is nothing to be done about it. The opposite of depression is not happiness, argues Solomon, it is vitality.

Chapter 8

Helping patients and relatives to live amidst dying

Chapter aims

After reading this chapter, you will be able to:

- understand how the different work associated with person-centred care combines to assist dying patients and their family members;
- draw together insights from preceding chapters to understand what within a passage of care might seem most individual, sensitive and supportive to families in difficult circumstances.

Introduction

This is the last of the case study chapters in this book and in it I bring together the different sorts of person-centred care work that you were introduced to in Chapter 2. The case study concerns a dying 11-year-old boy called Luke, his mother Sandra and Megan, the nurse who was his chief professional carer in the community. It is the most intimate of the case studies shared. Megan and I had met when I was a visiting lecturer at a hospice. I helped the students develop their reflective practice skills. After the teaching finished we stayed in touch and she sometimes asked my advice about coping with the care that she had to deliver on a daily basis. The emotional care work that she completed with families, and never more so than when the dying patient was a child, was at times taxing. Palliative care work with children and young adults teaches humility.

Nurses working in palliative care as elsewhere benefit from clinical supervision; the guidance and support of a mentor who helps the nurse to examine ideas about how care should be (normative), how care could be something that improves practice (formative), and which sustains the nurse as they deal with difficulties and uncertainties (restorative). In this case study I was a consultant friend rather than a clinical supervisor, but it is instructive to reflect on just how important such support is as nurses deal with complex and ambiguous issues. If we are to personalise care, to come closer to the patient as a person, just how is that done with due regard to professionalism, nurse confidence and development? Person-centred care is more exacting than care that relies upon a formula or a standard prescription. It is much more difficult to reflect in and on practice alone. Second and even third opinions may both improve service and sustain the nurse through taxing periods of patient care.

Megan explained that there was a patient that she was trying to help. Her first consultation with me related to body image issues but that later moved to something more about the young patient's relationship with his mother, Sandra. Luke had lost the power to smile, his facial expression was lopsided and he appeared to others as flat and emotionless. As Luke suffered from a brain stem glioma, one that was likely to prove fatal within the space of a year, it was probable that he would suffer other body image indignities. As Megan put it, Luke would feel his body crumbling and his mother would have to watch. While Megan was an expert in handling symptom control and especially pain management, she was struggling with some other psychological matters, those that make care seem more personal.

We agreed to talk regularly, the better to make sense of what she was trying to do to assist Luke and his mother Sandra. She had no need of assistance with the physical care that she delivered, but she would appreciate a sounding board as regards what she discussed with the family. As she put it, *when you get to dying, you can't escape what it means to be a person. That is what ends then. It's not the body, it's the sense of person that goes, unless you can leave that in the relatives' minds as a keepsake.*

Brain tumours and dying

While brain tumours arise in different parts of the brain and not all are malignant, they nonetheless account for 25 per cent of childhood cancer deaths in the UK (Rogers et al., 2016). Some 450 children are diagnosed with a brain tumour annually and, of those, 65 per cent survive for five or more years (Bennett et al., 2013). Of the brain tumours that do arise in children and young people, brain stem gliomas are the most aggressive with a median survival time of around nine months after diagnosis (Hassan et al., 2017). Fewer than one per cent of these patients live for five years. Brain stem gliomas (Diffuse Intrinsic Pontine Glioma (DIPG)) are typically treated with a six-week course of palliative radiotherapy. Because the tumour is intimately mixed with vital life-sustaining nerve pathways within the brain stem it is not amenable to surgery. Brain stem tumours rob parents of hope and they rapidly undermine the quality of life available to the young patient, often leaving them wheelchair-bound and with a variety of other communication and mobility difficulties.

Activity 8.1 Enquiry

Take a moment to view the YouTube video clip below concerning a 19-year-old young basketball player from Indiana, USA. Lauren Hill became a campaigner raising millions of dollars to aid brain tumour research. As you watch this video clip I would encourage you to reflect on two things:

1. Why leaving a legacy of research was important to Lauren and her mother.
2. How images of her before illness (playing basketball) and after illness (in a wheelchair struggling to speak) demonstrate the assault on her person.

Here is the web link: **www.youtube.com/watch?v=b8Jil0liOU4**

An outline answer is provided at the end of the chapter.

Dying poses a range of problems for nurses trying to deliver person-centred care. The first problem has already been alluded to, the sense of **personhood** soon to be lost, i.e., that which dignifies the existence of sentient (thinking) beings. If in health we can pretend to ourselves that death and dying are for another day, when a diagnosis of a terminal illness is made confrontation with death is impossible to avoid. Dependent on the nature of the illness and its trajectory (i.e., how rapidly it undermines physical and mental health functions), the patient is repeatedly reminded of their mortality and set almost daily challenges as regards living well (Barclay et al., 2014). Pain is often a problem that has to be countered, and here a balance has to be struck between sustaining a pain-free state and enabling the patient to remain alert and interactive enough to engage in activities that give them a sense of purpose (Thomas et al., 2018).

The challenges of dying

Dying poses a series of physical challenges that have to be overcome, for instance eating and drinking in a different way, urinating or defecating. There may be challenges associated with wound odour and deficits of mobility or communication, depending on the nature or the location of the disease (Campbell, 2014). The ability of the person to represent themselves through their body may become incrementally compromised (Hakanson and Ohlen, 2015). The body tells us that we are alive, through how we sense it, the way it feels, smells and functions. But a body damaged by disease and one with no real prospect of repair becomes a body that feels like a burden. Wellbeing is threatened by abnormal body experiences, those that signal that deterioration continues.

Dying itself, however, as a concept, poses its own difficulties. Distinctions are drawn (where possible) between the end of life (when death is imminent) and the more protracted business of dying that may extend over weeks or months. Because illness progresses at different paces, and because there may be exacerbations and comparative calm along the way, it is that much harder for nurses to negotiate care that suits needs (Mitchell et al., 2017). Dying is a dynamic process so, as well as trying to ascertain the needs and hopes of the patient, the nurse has to anticipate how these could change dependent on changes within the patient's body and their psychological efforts to cope with that. Megan said to me once, *anyone writing a book on care of the dying needs endless examples if it is to make sense.*

Person-centred care and dying

Where writers have written upon person-centred care of the dying patient, however, there are some recurring themes. Reed et al. (2017) described nurses' efforts to empower patients. A good quality of life was achieved where the nurse assisted patients to achieve a mixture of big and small personal goals. The small goals were often associated with quite discrete achievements: *I will get in the bath today, rather than have a blanket bath.* The big goals, however, were not necessarily those aspired to in health. Patients had to find new goals that related accurately to their felt energy levels and the limits imposed by an illness. Nurses who engaged in this work had to commit to it. Person-centred care couldn't be switched on and off, demonstrated more on some days than others, otherwise patients and relatives would feel cheated. The nurses had to get to know the patients and accept their quirks and foibles. Significantly, the nurses themselves had to feel supported. Megan secured assistance from hospice colleagues and management as well as from me.

Irrespective of the diagnosis of dying patients, other themes recurred. The first was establishing and sustaining a bond of trust. Patients feared abandonment precisely at a time when they knew they would have to let go: *I will have to let go, but please don't let go of me.* Hakanson et al. (2016) described the importance of this for very vulnerable homeless patients in Sweden. These patients, who already had dented dignity because of their lifestyle, needed additional assurance of their personal worth. The authors referred to this as *redignifying the person.*

In Germany, Strohbuecker et al. (2011) described the concerns of nurses and care home residents there. Residents wanted to be respected as a person and, to whatever degree it was possible, to retain a sense of personal control. That which defines 'adult' is the increased sense of control and agency to bring about change in personal life. Residents also wanted to retain contact with their family and the wider world and that sometimes meant that nurses had to help mediate how the patient seemed. Dying can be frightening for onlookers.

McGreevy (2015), writing about patients dying with dementia, highlighted the importance of carefully titrated medication. In the later stages of illness patients with dementia might become aggressive as well as disorientated. Still, it was important not to rely solely on antipsychotic medications to control challenging behaviours. Other psychological supports, such as art, music therapy, reminiscence, life story work and pet therapy could and should be used to help the patient retain dignity. The word dignity comes originally from the Latin term for coat-of-arms emblems that were displayed on medieval shields and banners (*dignitat-um*). They represented the honour and the station of the house of the bearer. In many senses the body too represents the honour of the self. So, when the body could not be relied upon to represent the self, it was important that other activities that were dignifying were deployed instead. When the body is despoiled, its image damaged beyond repair, then the patient may become stigmatised. Goffman's (2009) classic text *Stigma* was subtitled *Notes on the Management of Spoiled Identity.*

Writing about the ethics of palliative care, Furingsten et al. (2015) remind us that palliative care is not just about doing things to or for the patient (e.g., pain management), it is also about being with, attending and acting as a companion to the dying as well. In children this is especially taxing for nurses as care alternates between the parent and the professional carer. Nurses wonder how best to relate to patients, especially as the circumstances of the patient may deteriorate quite quickly. Attending a family involves reading what the parents and the child explain. It is about being different each day to suit the demands that arise there. It is unrealistic to be complacent about needs that can change in a moment. The nurse has to acknowledge the supreme injustice that a terminal illness represents for a child and their parents. The sense of sadness can seem overwhelming. No matter how expert the palliative care nurse becomes at managing physical problems, the psychological demands twist and turn before them in a bewildering series of ways.

Case study: Luke

As with some other neurological illnesses (see, for example, Chapter 3), Luke's illness started with a mix of confusing symptoms. He started to suffer severe headaches, often those that would awake him from sleep and which he described as *squeezing his head.* The fact that they woke Luke suddenly terrified him, causing him to scream in the middle of the night and bring Sandra rushing in. At 11 years of age Luke struggled to explain the headaches clearly. He linked them to bad dreams about school. Whether the dream caused the headache or vice versa, he was not sure, but he talked about the two as if they were one. As Luke started to exhibit some unsteadiness of gait, his mother was concerned. He seemed to bump into furniture frequently and sometimes said that he felt as though he might be sick, although Sandra had never seen Luke vomit. She began by conferring with his form teacher about his dreams, headaches and clumsiness and it was the teacher who urged her to take Luke to his GP as soon as possible. As far as the teacher was aware, Luke wasn't dealing with any personal problems at school. However, his handwriting had grown untidy and she wondered sometimes now whether Luke struggled to concentrate on his lessons.

The GP arranged for Luke to be referred to a neurologist and he, in turn, arranged a magnetic resonance imaging (MRI) scan. This revealed a large mass beneath his cerebrum and associated with structures running down into his brain stem. A brain stem glioma was diagnosed, something that devastated Sandra when she was told. However kindly the neurologist put it, the location of the tumour made it inoperable and therefore the right course of treatment would be radiotherapy. Sandra remembered that at that consultation she couldn't think straight and ask about prognosis. It was just important to start treatment and to counter the severe headaches, which were continuing. When their physician told her that the prognosis for these tumours was extremely poor Sandra was bereft: *How poor? Around a year,* said the doctor, taking her hand. He explained why they could not operate but that there was a team of nurses, excellent nurses, who could help Sandra.

That was how Sandra met Megan. Megan wasn't your run-of-the-mill nurse. She supported Portsmouth FC for one thing (that was Luke's assessment and he was a fervent supporter of the team). She also knew lots about chart music, something that Sandra never pretended to know. Luke and Megan began a friendship, one that wasn't entirely based on countering how sick and giddy he felt through radiotherapy, or upon the unsteady walking that continued to plague him. Under the effects of radiotherapy the tumour was shrinking, for now, and Luke's headaches seemed to abate. He felt relief that they were gone, although Megan insisted that, just in case, they should continue to monitor how he was feeling.

Seven months after the conclusion of the course of radiotherapy Luke relapsed. He had struggled with school work in the interim, feeling fatigued and dealing with the change in his appearance (alopecia). But now he started to collapse when he least expected it, on several occasions hitting his head when he fell. Luke struggled to speak for any length of time. He readily became breathless.

Sandra became panic-stricken. She chastised herself for daring to hope despite what the doctor had said. She criticised herself for becoming irritable with Luke after she

(Continued)

(Continued)

had struggled to sleep for fear of what might happen. Her conversations with Luke were difficult. She didn't want to tell him that he was getting worse and that he wouldn't be able to get better. For Sandra this amounted to confessing failure. If she had managed things better, somehow, she would have protected Luke. Now, she couldn't, she couldn't. There came a visit by Megan when Sandra snapped at her visitor.

You look after him, I can't! I don't know how to anymore!!

That morning, the atmosphere in the house was extremely tense. It sounded to Megan as if Sandra resented everything she did. Megan proceeded silently, caring for Luke until she could find something to say to Sandra upon leaving the house. Megan explained that she looked after Luke as regards his body and feeling comfortable. But she insisted that Sandra loved Luke. She had always loved Luke, that was evident and it was never in doubt. It was hard to watch someone so very ill, her baby, no matter how old Luke was. Sandra was allowed to hurt, allowed to shout, but, no, Megan would not give up on her either. *You come as a package Sandra, both together,* she insisted.

Hearing narratives

When Megan called me she confided that she had dealt with parental anger before but this time Sandra's rage seemed especially visceral. Sandra felt utterly forlorn. She didn't know what she could do. She couldn't make Luke better. She couldn't be an expert with drugs. She couldn't stop Luke feeling terror at what was going to befall him. Sandra felt purposeless. There was nothing that she could think of to do that would seem enough. In sharp contrast to the gradually extracted narrative of the patient Ted in Chapter 7, Sandra's narrative exploded from her in bouts of dismay. The sheer force of her accounts, their sudden exasperated introduction into conversations, made it extremely hard for Megan to follow them. Sometimes narratives are shared with extreme emotion, even venom.

I need you to tell me that I'm right ... about what I've heard, Megan said to me.

Her summary seemed sound. Given the detailed way she had described Sandra's despairing outburst, I couldn't imagine another way to explain the mother's angst. We talked about that. There were other contextual influences that I didn't yet know about. It was as if Sandra had howled and a howl didn't specify needs. It was simply raw hurt.

What about Luke I wondered? How much does he understand about his illness? He is 11, an age when more abstract reasoning starts to become possible (Cowie, 2012). A child on the cusp of adolescence begins to imagine futures, to conceive of progress or the lack of it, over time. Equally importantly, I wondered, what had Sandra, or Megan, told Luke about his illness? Had either of them admitted that he wouldn't be able to get better, that he would die? Megan knew about discussions about death, the theory of the matter and ways to explore how to prepare for that. Megan was ready to talk about death if Luke asked. But Luke was 11 and Sandra was alone (she and her husband had divorced, the father was estranged and unwilling to become *involved again for the wrong reasons*). Talking for Luke and Sandra was probably much more complicated. They had each other and dying perhaps sounded like another abandonment.

I don't think that Sandra has admitted that to Luke, Megan said, *she thinks that she has to be strong for him. It's a day at a time for Sandra, a day at a time, dealing with each difficulty as it comes up. But she feels so disheartened because she keeps needing to ask my help. That's why she snapped at me.*

I asked Megan about the care measures that she engaged in. There was the monitoring; the checking of Luke's vision and his coordination. A wheelchair had been secured as he was so unsteady on his feet. Megan was assisting with oral hygiene because Luke was struggling to control his mouth in the usual way. He could speak, but only in short sentences.

What is Sandra doing? I asked.

Watching him die, replied Megan. *That's how she sees it.*

We returned to Luke and how he spoke about his illness. Megan described how he was *being a little soldier.* I thought I knew about that, but I asked anyway. *What does that involve? Well* (and Megan found this difficult),

When his mum is there, he doesn't complain. He might point for a tissue for his mouth. He will signal when he needs the toilet, but there is no complaint with it. When his mum is out of the room he groans or grimaces more. It's like he can't hide it then.

I said, *you're the secret witness.*

Yes, she said.

And that's exhausting, I ventured.

Yes, she said.

Activity 8.2   Critical thinking

What do you think is critically important about the communication between Luke and his mother? Why is that perhaps so influential as regards person-centred care?

An outline answer is provided at the end of the chapter.

Anticipating the concerns, needs and requirements of the patient

In this part of the case study chapters I usually discuss the prior research, audit and experience-reviewing work that the nurse has done and which is used strategically to manage care in a sensitive way. On this occasion though, Megan and I were stuck. She had a wealth of knowledge relating to symptom management, to the explanation of dying trajectories and the preparation of relatives for a time when a loved one was no longer there. None of the familiar evidence, however, seemed right to use at this stage. To instruct Sandra on what dying involves would seem trite in the extreme.

Megan: *I want to help Sandra feel better.*

Bob: *You're right. She's lost to Luke right now. She doesn't know how to help him.*

Megan: *I don't know what to say to her about telling Luke what the future is. I've been in the library and read stuff, but it all feels formula. They're talking and not talking. They're hinting to one another and stepping away again.*

Bob: *How long do you imagine that we have?*

Megan: *Before Luke dies?*

Bob: *Yes, as far as you can guess .... I know it's a guess, but if you can't do everything, then what you do has to be the best.*

Megan: *I can't guess! I can't.*

Bob: *We have to speculate ... it has to be something that Sandra can do in time. It has to feel the best use of time.*

Megan: *Two months, maybe two months.*

Two months seemed insufficient time for Megan to search afresh. I said that I would look as I had access to additional libraries and I would look for ways to describe the problem and find something that might make sense for Sandra. If Megan telephoned me in a week's time I might have something to offer. But she would have to judge it. She would have to decide whether she could use it.

Sharing risks and identifying desirable ways forward

It is debatable whether any professional can confidently offer help when they understand the clinical problem at a distance. But, against that, there is a counter-argument that sometimes a mind once removed can see issues from a fresh angle. So I started searching articles on person-centred care and the dying. I searched in particular for articles relating to children. As far as I could ascertain from Megan, there were two related problems.

1. Sandra felt disempowered. She couldn't fulfil her normal parenting role because (she believed) Luke was now a patient and Megan was the perceived expert. It was as if Luke had been handed over in despair.

2. Communication between son and mother was ambiguous. No one seemed sure about whether to talk about dying. No matter what might be said to Sandra as regards child cognitive development and ability to reason dying, she seemed unsure whether she could tell Luke. For her to do so could be to acknowledge despair.

Two philosophical papers

I worked quickly on the search. The evidence had to be a servant. It had to suit a need. I found two papers that might help us, but neither in their standard unadjusted form. This was the problem with evidence, it was abstract. It wasn't like a recipe with instructions on how to mix the ingredients. Goodness, I thought, you're thinking in analogies all the time. But that seemed to be what it sometimes took. Perhaps the problem can be seen this way? What if the issue is really like this? When I thought about it, academics and researchers offered more and more information, more explanations, but there was always the need to interpret and to apply. There was always the need for something to bridge matters.

The first paper had been written in a philosophy journal by a group of authors who acknowledged that person-centred care was implicit in palliative care, but that it rarely found a practical expression, save for attention to symptom management (Ohlen et al., 2017). No one talked about the person as that was too vague in times of patient/ relative distress. The authors described the usual attributes of person-centred care (see Chapter 1), but what struck me most was a short passage within the article about how people express their self. It described things that had the potential to make a person feel whole. Ohlen et al. (2017) described it in four terms.

1. Activities (there are things that we do and others help us do that express our life, a feeling of integrity. These are subverted in terminal illness but they need not be extinguished).

2. Narratives (we tell stories to ourselves about who we are, what we are doing, and why that matters. It was one of the key prompts for this book).

3. We demonstrate skills (those that we own that might set us apart).

4. We exercise powers (often role-related. Power while dying is diminished but new powers might emerge. A dying person could console).

The second paper was also philosophical and it examined the reasoning and the morality of dying children (Hoffmaster, 2011). This paper reported at some length on the earlier work of an author who had studied how children reasoned about dying (Bluebond-Langner, 1978). I could have kicked myself for not remembering this work, which I had read while studying sociology. Children had their own form of reasoning through illness and treatment events that was not classically rational, but which could mean that our fears about talking to them about dying were more pronounced than they need be. Bluebond-Langner (1978) explained that children with leukaemia discerned how poorly they were through several strategies.

- Dedicated watching (they checked how children with different illnesses were treated and how much time medical staff spent with them. This helped determine how ill someone was).
- Reasoning methods (children deduced things from their observations, for example, if you were excused lessons/schooling in hospital and you were known to have a serious illness, then that might mean staff thought your time was limited).
- Creative construction (children pretended to be asleep so that they could listen to adult-to-adult conversations. This enabled them to piece together information that might not have been otherwise forthcoming).
- Critical assessment of their deductions (they talked to each other about what they had noticed).

Activity 8.3 Speculating

Can you guess why these two papers might seem valuable as regards Sandra and Luke? Jot down your ideas before reading on.

As this is based on your own reflections there is no sample answer provided at the end of the chapter. However, some thoughts are offered in the following dialogue.

I telephoned Megan with some 'what if' ideas. I didn't know whether these could work. I didn't know whether they would seem worthwhile.

Bob: *I've found this article and in some ways it is so obvious. It may seem stupid, so common sense as not worth talking about.*

Megan: *You haven't described it yet, let me decide.*

Bob: *OK. Sandra feels useless, but what if you can convince her that what makes any of us, even an 11-year-old, feel individual, feel loved, is if she helps with things that are really close to who they think they are, what they are most passionate about. What if you give Sandra a framework to think about her work?*

Megan: *It sounds abstract.*

Bob: *We feel human, individual, because of our activities, our skills and narratives. You know, the stories we tell ourselves.*

Megan: *How does that work for Sandra?*

Bob: *Well, she sees Luke as dying right? He's dying in her heart, because it hurts so much. He can't be living if he is dying, that is maybe how she sees it. He's not doing living things because there can be no long-term outcome. Everything she has done with him has been about growing up and being a great adult. She doesn't believe that she's allowed to do those things with Luke anymore.*

Megan: *She's waiting for him to die.*

Bob: *Yes. So what makes for dignity? What makes us feel proud of ourselves? We do things despite the challenges. So now there is work for Sandra to do that focusses on Luke's living, however that is possible given his health.*

Megan: *For example …?*

Bob: *Portsmouth FC, what do you know about it?*

Megan: *The agony and the ecstasy!* (She laughs.)

Bob: *I know. But, joking apart, what does Luke know about his football club?*

Megan: *Everything … absolutely everything!*

Bob: *So maybe Luke needs to teach Sandra about Portsmouth FC. So maybe Sandra needs to show Luke that she needs his knowledge? So maybe Sandra needs to be a learner rather than a protector because she then sees how much pleasure that could give Luke? It's nothing to do with illness, or cancer, or dying, it's talking about living.*

Megan: *I know nothing about Portsmouth FC.*

Bob: *Exactly, you know nothing. Make sure that Luke does the teaching.*

We moved on. What skills did Luke retain that Sandra could help with while Megan *did the technical bits of care.* Luke could draw. There were pictures of animals in his bedroom. Megan didn't know whether Sandra could draw but she was going to be persuaded to try. While they did that, it would be a good idea to recount memories, stories about visits to the zoo, safari park, whatever they had ever shared. We didn't know whether that would work. It was really very simple. Megan was going to give Sandra work to do. That the work, if it succeeded, might add dignity to dying now and happier memories afterwards was a theory that could be explained in full as time went by. For now, Megan hoped to get 'buy in' to the idea from Sandra.

Bob: *Another paper I read and forgot about. There is this researcher who did a lot of great work with children suffering from leukaemia, especially those who had gone through the first treatments and were now on palliative care measures. She researched how children worked out their prognosis, even quite young children. I'll email you the reference.*

Megan: *How do they do it then?*

I described what you have read above.

Megan: *Luke knows but he's protecting his mum.*

Bob: *I don't know, do you think so?*

Megan: *Yes, I suspect that he does. He cloaks his pains and aches from her. He shares them with me instead.*

Bob: *I don't know why Luke pretends not to know, if that's what's happening. They might simply be terrified, together in their own little spaces ....*

Megan: *But it could mean that they love one another ....*

Bob: *Yes ....*

Megan: *But using that now? How can I use it to help them?*

Bob: *Have another guess.*

Megan: *If I asked Luke what he thought was about to happen? If I asked him if he wanted to tell his mum things ....*

Bob: *Or to be an ally. What if you asked him whether he wanted your help to protect his mum? I know that we usually think open is honest and best. But what if they usually cope by protecting each other. What if this is what enables Luke to feel that he is loving his mum?*

Megan: *That's dangerous, in practice, it's a secret.*

Bob: *I know. But if you're already helping Sandra to give something to Luke ....*

Megan: *I'll have to ponder it.*

Bob: *Yes. It's a theory. Theory means little without context.*

Agreeing roles and what counts as progress

By her own admission, Sandra was feeling increasingly as if she had no role left other than to watch her son suffer. To witness deterioration, to offer a warm presence, was certainly important, but it didn't feel constructive to Sandra. She described to Megan how, after her husband had left her, she had busied herself trying to be the *complete parent* to Luke. If he didn't have a role-model father then he would have a role-model mother. It was on a Friday morning that Megan visited the family and, before starting her usual checks with Luke, she suggested that she had some work for Sandra to do. At first the idea of work being assigned seemed like an imposition but Megan insisted that it had a scientific and a human purpose. The 'scientists' (it seemed better than 'philosophers' Megan said) had realised that people felt more dignified when they were assisted to do particular self-defining things. So the logical work was to ascertain what those were for Luke and to concentrate on those. Football was the obvious starting point. Sandra was going to have to become very interested in Luke's favourite football team. Megan also suggested that they draw together. Sandra explained that she could draw horses but, as to her skills with any other animal, well, that was limited.

Please try, suggested Megan, *let Luke talk about how much better he is at it than you. Let him talk about any memories that you have together that link to it.*

Sandra guessed that it was about building memories.

You're suggesting this for me too, Sandra challenged.

I don't have memories with Luke, that's your contribution. Only you can make him feel good that way. But it's not just about making a memory box. If you're waiting for Luke to die, then you don't help him to live. Luke can do both and maybe you have to show him that? Megan responded.

A week later Megan shared her reflections with me again. The work assignment had been successful. For sure Luke got tired, so the chats about football and the drawing had to work with his energy limits, but it was making Sandra feel a good deal more useful. I asked whether Luke seemed to be enjoying it and apparently he was. His mum's football knowledge was *rubbish, but she can only improve.* I wondered what Megan thought would count as progress, was it solely to do with the amount of time that Luke and his mum did activities together? She assured me that, no, it was going to be judged by *how few times I get a frosty reception when I visit.* She laughed. She was right too. Sometimes a measure of progress fuels the nurse as well. She couldn't do this work without that.

We talked then about the second idea, asking Luke about his illness and ascertaining how much he understood and whether he was protecting his mother. Megan had decided to reserve that idea though. Here is an extract of her impeccable reasoning.

Now that Luke and Sandra have more things to do together, things that aren't just about his illness, they might start to talk about cancer and dying. Luke might be ready and Sandra might feel able to let Luke lead on that. We assume that parents must always lead, but dying patients, even little ones, are sometimes wise. They might have to lead. If they don't talk, if they keep that work together in another place, I can always try to see what Luke knows later. We can use your idea as a plan B.

Candidly, I wished that I had thought about that. The two elements of care were interlinked. Success in one might obviate the need for the other, and with it the risks of the kindly subterfuge of Megan allying herself with Luke to manage his secret and forestall his mother's pain.

Activity 8.4 Evaluating

Look back now and jot down some ideas about how Megan and I worked together to try and find something that assisted Sandra. We each did different sorts of work. What does that suggest about person-centred care planning? What does it suggest to you about the relationship between person-centred care and evidence-based practice?

An outline answer is provided at the end of the chapter.

Learning lessons and adjusting plans for the future

My conversations with Megan over the next few weeks became rather more sporadic and mixed with feelings of sadness and relief. Megan reported that Luke's condition was rapidly deteriorating and that the early drawings that he had done with Sandra were now much less accomplished. Sandra showed them to Megan and cried, comparing the drawings that she had dated on the back so that she could see her loss. She refused to cry in front of Luke, feeling that she must be strong. However, she had done several things that gave them both pleasure. Old football programmes and some DVD coverage of Portsmouth FC matches had been bought. Some of the matches they watched over and over again. Megan felt very welcome in the home, carrying out her physical care activities, keeping Luke's mouth and skin clean. She felt able to discuss with Sandra how to provide fluids and nutrients to Luke in a way that enabled him to avoid pressure sores. They agreed that the goal was not *to build Luke up* but to *stop his skin breaking down*. So fluid and nutrient intake was managed against what Luke felt he could manage. Luke slept for increasingly longer periods.

I asked whether Luke or Sandra had confided in each other, whether they had shared new conversations about what was happening? They hadn't. The 'living' conversations and activities had continued as before, talking about football, watching football and, more recently still, feeding birds from the living-room window. Luke was content for his mum to teach him the differences between cock and hen chaffinches, and to show him how much bigger a bullfinch was. Sandra had wished that she had taught him these things earlier. She said that he seemed so little when she explained the details. He wasn't 11 anymore, he felt six or so. Megan asked whether Sandra thought that he was humouring her, showing an interest in bird watching that he barely felt. Sandra was unsure, but she was grateful that he stuck with it. You never knew which birds would come to the table.

Messages

Megan related something that moved me.

Megan: *Do you remember that you told me about the American girl, Lauren Hill, the basketball player who died of brain stem glioma?*

I had remembered. I'd offered it to her not because I thought it could teach Megan about palliative care, but because, in the video clip, the mother of Laura had looked so supportive. I hoped that it would encourage Megan.

Megan: *Well, yesterday, Luke gave me one of his mum's bird identification books. He'd hidden it under the mattress of his bed. He made me open the page on the bullfinch and there was one of his drawings inside. It was a bit squiggly but it was definitely the bullfinch.*

Bob: *Brilliant … that's brilliant. A gift. Did he want you to give it to her?*

Megan: *When he had gone, he told me. When he had gone to play football. He'd written on it, 'I know mum. Please don't cry, I love you.'*

Lauren Hill had left notes around the house for her parents too. They described all that she knew and feared and how she felt about them both. They found them again and again hidden in different cubby holes after she had died.

I don't know whether Megan and Luke should have had the conversation about what she suspected that he understood and why he acted the *brave soldier*. It might have helped and Megan might have been able to comfort him some more as he dealt with what dying meant. She might have been able to relate the conversations to Sandra at a time that Luke permitted. But I doubt that it would have been more eloquent or consoling than a note in a book about birds. Luke wanted his mum to find it sticking out of the book afterwards.

Three days later Luke died. It was in his sleep and Sandra found him the next morning. Megan admitted that she returned to the house to make sure that the book and the picture had been found. They had been.

Person-centred care insights

Sometimes care is felt isn't it. You cannot nurse without that. If it is personal it engages the emotions as well as our powers of reasoning. It would have been much harder to relate this particular case study to you in other than the more intimate dialogue terms. I want you to sense the feeling involved with it, the fervent search for information that might help, the wisdom of the experienced palliative care practitioner and the pleasure in an outcome that seemed to offer a sense of closure, despite the very challenging circumstances of Luke's illness. Sometimes person-centred care feels like a discovery. There comes a time when care that is person-centred is intuitively judged and beyond usual scrutiny about what principles applied or didn't apply.

Contact time and individual caring

But I should try to make some points. The first thing to say is that it seems to me that only in protracted care relationships, those where the nurse has a pivotal role to play, can you be assured that all the different sorts of person-centred care work (Chapter 2) will be evidenced. Shorter periods of care, care where continuity is fractured by many referrals and movement of the patient, admit fewer opportunities for us to join up the dots and make the care seem perfect. In acute care, with a more passing contact, the person-centred care is perhaps much more about attending and communicating. It is about conveying an interest and a sense of concern. It is about adjusting care subtly rather than fashioning care entirely around the patient. Such person-centred care is no less valuable for that. Nurses work within the constraints of the time shared with the patient, the opportunities afforded to get to know them as an individual. Compassionate care finds what's available and uses it to help.

In more protracted care relationships, however, and perhaps quintessentially in care of dying patients and their families, there is a chance to join up the different elements of person-centred care work. We all die individually but we need not die feeling alone if care has been well arranged. In this instance, Megan has moved to orchestrate care in a way that worked to the benefit of Luke and his mother. She has found ways to help them to demonstrate love for each other. It is perhaps doubtful that Sandra could ever have comfortably been honest with Luke about what was happening. It was simply too painful. Her formula was to stay silent to be strong, to think of Luke rather than herself. Megan gave her some tools to do that with. Sandra was given some new work to do, that which was mutually sustaining for her son and herself.

Working with the clients' agendas

Person-centred care works with the patients' or the carers' agenda. However satisfying or perhaps useful it might have been to promote a more open discussion about dying and death, Megan worked with what Sandra and (I think) what Luke wanted. She introduced ideas to Sandra and then carefully watched how they were used. It was as real as an injection, as relevant as a painkiller. Megan was a meticulous and a skilful practitioner who quickly grasped what a tool could do and then made sure that it operated properly in the patient context.

In the end there was no need to help Luke with communication. He had proven every bit as inquisitive, reasoning and caring as the children in Bluebond-Langner's (1978) study. Luke seems to have sensed what his mum needed and decided to give that to her, managing his dying in different ways, sometimes honest and open with Megan and then cloaked with his mum. I asked Megan how she had decided to hold off the insights conversation with Luke and whether this was all to do with watching how the other 'living' work proceeded. This is what she said to me:

> *I remember when I stopped believing in Santa as a guy who came down a chimney and began thinking of him as a symbol for parents who planted warmth in your heart. I saw how much pleasure my parents got in pretending. It meant that they kept some magic in the world for us.*

Luke and Sandra wanted to pretend. Megan facilitated that. That Luke at the very end signalled to Megan that he knew what was happening also confirmed what he was trying to do. He was 11 years old approaching 80.

Mixing up the person-centred care roles

In Table 2.1 of Chapter 2 (page 34) you were introduced to some of the person-centred care roles that nurses often fulfil. At least three of those were employed in this case study and by two nurses working together. Both Megan and I acted as problem analysts. It is rather doubtful whether that would have been so easy if one nurse worked alone. In the end it took two nurses to explore a nuanced problem, one acting as the information searcher and the other as the ideas applier. Person-centred nursing care is often like that. It involves collaboration, that which analyses a problem and which assures the nurse in their work.

Megan acted as a counsellor/advisor to Sandra and assisted her to believe that she had an active role to play. That which purposefully comforted Luke now might, in the years to come, assist Sandra to grieve for the loss of her son. Person-centred care pays dividends, sometimes ones that present long down the road. Person-centred care is a wise investment, that which sustains patients, carers and the reputation of nursing as well.

Megan was also a confidant to both Sandra and her son Luke. I wonder how comfortable you feel with the discussion of a secret preserved, a problem handled in an indirect fashion? Sometimes, that which is most personal, most person-centred, is that which deals with issues in the patient's or lay carer's own way. It might not seem the most comfortable approach to you, but if you help sustain the patient/lay carer, to help them feel that they coped, cared and shared in ways that were personally sustainable, you may have done some of the best work.

Chapter summary

Caring for dying patients and their families represents the quintessential person-centred-care challenge. As the person dies so the notion of person, of self, is threatened. That which we have felt proud about as regards our body, its function and integrity, is undermined. Achievements that marked us out will have gone, save for in the record and memory of others. The pace and pattern of illness casts doubt on what we can be sure about anymore. The lay carer may often feel bereft, witnessing decline but wondering what they can do to alleviate suffering during the dying process. Nurses working in palliative care are accustomed to helping patients to prepare more positive memories to help counter grief after the patient has died, but they may be less sure-footed as regards helping the relative to play a collegiate role while the patient dies. There is a risk that first one cares and then the other, each respectful of the other but not necessarily as well co-ordinated as they might be.

- Anticipating needs and requirements in palliative care has to address both the patient and any lay carer. Sometimes, at best, the nurse's measure to help the one helps both.
- Evidence associated with palliative care might not always be the right fit. Because dying is so individual and patient circumstances so varied, the nurse might have to search afresh for new elements of evidence to help solve problems. Sometimes the evidence comes from unusual places.

(Continued)

(Continued)

- Person-centred care in the palliative care context is often consultative. The emotional work of supporting a patient and family can seem overwhelming. There is also often value in consulting with others to understand a need or a problem in a new way.

- Person-centred care in palliative care settings involves some subtle orchestration. The nurse suggests ideas, offers tools, makes facilities available. In many cases, though, it is the patient or lay carer that dictates what will be used to greatest effect.

Activities: Brief outline answers

Activity 8.1   Enquiry (p144)

1. I think it likely that, as well as the obvious hoped-for benefits to other patients diagnosed with a devastating illness, the psychology merit of this work for Lauren and her family was that they made something positive out of a negative. Brain stem glioma, in terms of accumulating physical deficits, feels like a continuous rear-guard action, one that exhausts and undermines morale continuously. So Lauren leaves a legacy, not only of funds but resilient attitude in the face of adversity, one that perhaps brought comfort to her family over the ensuing years.

2. The video clip offers a sharp contrast between Lauren's physical appearance before and after illness and treatment. Not only was Lauren extremely active before her illness, but her body posture and movement signals freedom. To be confined to a wheelchair, to struggle to speak and to facially express your emotions and experiences, highlights how an illness traps you inside a body that causes pain and distress. I think that it's worth considering the bravery required to manage a public celebrity image when physical function and appearance are incrementally undermined. Appearance is used to further a heartfelt cause. Lauren managed this at a time in life when body image is usually central to the person's identity.

Activity 8.2   Critical thinking (p149)

One of the ways in which people cooperate to best effect is in problem solving. It's difficult, however, to liaise when the problem isn't named. Each individual may have complex reasons for not talking about something that is at the centre of their mutual difficulties. To expose those difficulties through raising a conversation about death may seem overwhelming. So the carer and the patient tackle other, more minor, superficial issues. They implicitly agree to set aside the unspeakable challenge before them. One of the risks associated with this is that either patient or carer brew emotional problems so large that they are damaged psychologically. For the carer, there is the risk that they might blame themselves for perceived shortfalls in care or loving over the longer term. Sometimes people need to talk, to express the emotions they harbour so deeply (catharsis). Facilitating that, though, is extremely hard for any nurse to do, both with regard to choosing the right time and place, and thereafter with regard to managing the rehearsal of memories, emotions and fears that follow.

Caring for patients and carers in such circumstances can feel like managing a pressure cooker. You are unsure whether the preferred communication approach can be sustained. What if emotions suddenly erupt? Might a very vulnerable patient lose their most important carer?

Communication difficulties such as this are nearly always deep-seated and woven into the relationship history. Megan cannot know all that Luke signifies to Sandra and vice versa. She learns about their relationship piecemeal and incrementally. The problem is that many useful support measures might depend on what patient and lay carer feel able to talk about. Much that is therapeutic during dying concerns words as well as actions. To act in a person-centred way, Megan has to understand the person and the relationship. It can be a little like making a jigsaw puzzle when the picture has been lost (another analogy I know). Megan has to think on her feet, and no matter what she has been taught or has gleaned from experience, reflection in action is always harder to use with confidence. She has to speculate.

Activity 8.4   Evaluating (p155)

There was a division of labour, wasn't there? We worked using our different strengths. Megan is the palliative care expert. I knew how to translate ideas into possible actions. Because I wasn't having to reflect in action, only on action, I had something additional to offer Megan as help. Neither of those elements of work would have been much use without the other. Sometimes it takes a friend to help a practitioner facing a conundrum and sometimes it takes the brakes of the practitioner to counter a too-flamboyant idea of the friend. Person-centred care (I believe) is often about such collaborations. It is about 'what if' thinking and a willingness to ask questions about what has seemed obvious. Nurses need to speculate. The most important part of that here related to the possibility that Sandra's grief had robbed her of what she might normally have done, i.e., to have helped Luke with things that made life seem worth living. After all, what demanded that you couldn't talk about football or drawing up to the last breath that you took?

The use of evidence here is worth some extra thought. In many instances the person-centred carer accrues evidence and other forms of information to use strategically as needed. But clearly there are times when there is not enough evidence or the right evidence. Sometimes we need to look again. But the searching is different. It's not a search for that which *should be* done, it is a search for that which *could be* done. Evidence has to serve a purpose. Perhaps after writing nursing essays this seems surprising. So often we use references to justify action. It's considered inappropriate to make assertions unless 'it is backed up by evidence'. But practice rarely works so neatly. We develop hunches about need, we start to formulate possible explanations and then we search for evidence that might help. Speculation remains a recurring skill within person-centred care.

Further reading

Fersko-Weiss, H (2017) *Caring for the Dying: The Doula Approach to a Meaningful Death.* London: Orion Spring.

There is no formula for supporting a dying person, but this is an interesting read as it covers how we talk about dying and death. Chapter 4 deals with truth-telling, Chapter 5 with active listening and Chapter 7 with legacy projects. All of these resonate with the case study in this chapter and for nurses interested in person-centred care.

McCartney, M (2014) *Living with Dying: Finding Care and Compassion at the End of Life.* London: Pinter and Martin.

Margaret McCartney writes in a refreshingly direct and practical manner about a subject that a lot of fellow GPs meet, looking after patients who die in the community. She is forthright in dealing with the politics of dying, with the fears that clinicians have and why those can lead to an over-reliance on medication. The discussion of what counts as a quality death is particularly good.

Useful websites

www.nationalvoices.org.uk/blogs/person-centred-care-2017-what-about-end-life

Riley, L (2017) *Person-Centred Care in 2017: What About at the End of Life?* Research officer: Compassion for Dying, National Voices. National Voices is a coalition of British healthcare charities for promoting the wellbeing of patients. Person-centred care is a recurring theme in their lobbying work, so it is interesting to start with this blog page on end-of-life care and to explore outwards using the links within it. National Voices presented their report on *Person-Centred Care* in 2017 and that can be reached from a hyperlink here.

endoflifecareamibitions.org.uk/…/Ambitions-for-Palliative-and-End-of-Life-Care.pdf

National Palliative and End of Life Care Partnership: *Ambitions for Palliative and End of Life Care: A National Framework for Local Action 2015–2020.* This partnership is made up of a wide variety of government and related care agencies in the UK, who have set out their ambitions for palliative care in this document. Significantly, person-centred care features strongly. It's valuable to read these ambitions and then, as we approach the end of the target period, to reflect on whether ambitions have been realised. See what you think.

Chapter 9 Looking forward to the future

NMC Standards of Proficiency for Registered Nurses

This chapter will address the following platforms and proficiencies:

Platform 1: Being an accountable professional

At the point of registration, the registered nurse will be able to:

1.13 demonstrate the skills and abilities required to develop, manage and maintain appropriate relationships with people, their families, carers and colleagues.

1.19 act as an ambassador, upholding the reputation of your profession, and promoting public confidence in nursing, health and care services.

Chapter aims

After reading this chapter, you will be able to:

- demonstrate awareness of the outstanding challenges and opportunities that lie ahead for person-centred care in the future;
- review the benefits for nurses of a pragmatic, carefully focussed approach to person-centred care in a stressful working environment.

Introduction

In the final chapter of this book I summarise the key responsibilities of the nurse and relate these to the contextual factors that pose challenges if person-centred care is to succeed in the future. This is no mean feat for the issues affecting healthcare in general and the work of nurses in particular are complex. Nursing work is only one element of a healthcare service, however it is one that could prove vital if person-centred care was arranged imaginatively in the future. To set the scene for this chapter I want to make three opening arguments to you. Each of these has an impact on what the future of person-centred care might look like and what the nurse is then able to achieve.

1. Nursing has begun to slowly clarify what it means by person-centred care, but further work is needed. While in the past much of that has been idealistic and without adequate concern for scarce resources, this book makes the case for more focussed, modest, but helpful interventions that can significantly improve the lives of patients. To discuss this I will be returning to the sorts of pragmatic person-centred care work that you first read about in Chapter 2. Best practice person-centred care relies on understanding which care work we do, when and why. The key question here will be, what does it take to demonstrate person-centred care in the most effective and efficient way?

2. How people think of health and healthcare affects to a significant degree what we can achieve. If the patient's conception of health and their role as a patient differs from that of healthcare staff then person-centred care becomes much more difficult. My argument is that person-centred care has the greatest chance of success where patients and nurses have similar ideas of what their partnership entails and what it is working towards. The key question here then is, what can or should be expected of care partnerships?

3. Person-centred care needs to be professionally fulfilling as well as delivering a good service. This may surprise you as we are more used to focussing on the patient and their needs. In person-centred care, it is important to sustain your belief and commitment. I argue that unless there are professional rewards within person-centred care for you, i.e., a satisfaction in your work, best practice is difficult to sustain. Person-centred care could become a mantra about what *should* be rather than about what *can* be. The key question here then is, what about person-centred care might best sustain your satisfaction in care delivery?

What does it take to implement person-centred care in the most effective and efficient way?

In Chapter 2 of this book you read about five types of person-centred care work, which I suggested represent a realistic care approach within a healthcare service where resources are limited. The five types of person-centred care work were:

1. anticipating concerns, needs and requirements;
2. hearing the narratives of patients and others;
3. sharing risks and identifying ways forward;
4. agreeing roles and what counts as progress;
5. learning lessons and adjusting future plans.

The case studies within this book have illustrated those types of care work in action. The work within the first case study, Chapter 3, was relatively discrete and focussed (helping a patient with an impending multiple sclerosis diagnosis). You might have considered it to be quite minor, something that was little more than common sense and a proper human concern for the feelings of another person. As the case studies have built one on another, however, the complexity of the care work has increased and it has often involved more than one type of work. Work associated with sharing and managing risks, agreeing roles and learning lessons develop in stages after the first evidence use and narrative-hearing work has begun. More complex person-centred care work is increasingly dependent on partnership and, even among the case studies discussed in this book, that was not always straightforward. Successful person-centred care has required communication between different healthcare professionals. Time spent earlier on, however, has often enabled a valuable saving afterwards as there has been less chance of recurring health problems and a reduced risk of complications later on. You may have noted this investment element of care work at play in the case studies relating to a patient with bowel cancer, assistance to a depressed pensioner and the care afforded to a dying boy and his mother. Significantly, the work has involved rather more staff time, and that is costly, but it has not necessarily involved the use of additional materials. Often person-centred care makes the very best use of existing resources, rather than demanding the development of additional ones.

Implementing successful person-centred care involves doing the right work at the right time. Preparation can save time and work when the patient arrives. It can also help limit the need for corrective work much later on. There is value in coming to understand a given clientele really well, so that you can research their experiences and needs with authority, and anticipate what may be required by patients. Where nurses work in a multitude of different settings, with different client groups (for instance working as an agency nurse) it is much harder to practise in a person-centred-care way. This is precisely because it is harder for you to anticipate patient care needs. If you move your care location regularly, it is unrealistic to research the relevant patient experience of illness, coping and patient support in ways that you can present as intuitive, knowledgeable and sensitive to the next patient met. Some degree of client-group specialism is likely to help you better implement person-centred care.

Anticipating patient concerns, needs and requirements involves being extremely well-informed about the client group of patients. It involves accessing, collating and sometimes completing research with colleagues yourself, to better understand the patient experience. What you learn about research, especially that relating to the patient's experience of illness and treatment, will benefit you in the future. Some areas of patient experience are very well-served by research, for instance in cancer care and chronic illnesses, but in other areas there may well be gaps where, for the time being, you will need to draw more heavily upon local care audit data, patient feedback and case studies of patients that you have known. Accessing, reading and understanding research and other data are vital to becoming a confident and authoritative person-centred care nurse.

Collecting and using patient experience evidence to support best practice in future care is vital. We require not only evidence of the patient experience of illness but of treatment and support too. If person-centred care works closely with patient percep-tions then we need research on the patient perspectives relating to all elements of care. What is it like to undergo diagnostic tests? What are the key needs while diagnosis is awaited? What does it feel like to be presented with different treatment options?

You perhaps noticed how prominent securing, hearing and understanding patient and lay carer narratives was within the case studies. We need to understand the nar-ratives of both the patient and their partner when a patient suffers a heart attack and rehabilitation depends on both people trusting the recommended course of action (Chapter 6). Using relevant evidence to anticipate patient care concerns and requirements, and combining that with a thorough grasp of narratives, is at the heart of effective person-centred care. Patients are much more likely to share their narra-tive with us when we have asked questions that signal that we understand common problems encountered with their illness, those that they have encountered too. The questions that we ask focus on particular issues that the patient is most likely to have already encountered. We establish a rapport when the patient feels that we quickly understand their circumstances.

However, eliciting patient narratives is not easy and sometimes we cannot expect to obtain all that we need to know in one conversation. We need to return again and again to patient experience as this can change rapidly. *How are you feeling today?* becomes a professional enquiry and one that we build on, rather than a social pleas-antry. To encourage patients to talk candidly we have to assure them places of privacy and to be honest about how we will use the information that they share with us. Trust is important. While eliciting patient narratives relies on some skills (e.g., asking open questions, attending to what is said, summarising what you understand), it also relies on foreknowledge of what may likely be of concern to patients sharing a diagnosis. What we ask about is as important as how we ask questions, as well as setting an envi-ronment so patients feel able to confide thoughts.

Gathering and using evidence to best effect, combined with a sincere and professional interest in the narratives of patients and lay carers, forms a foundation for the other areas of pragmatic person-centred care. From what patients tell us about their experi-ences and hopes we start to understand what risks concern them. These might or might not be the same as the clinical risks that we know are associated with a particular illness, disease or disability. We start to learn what they think that the care process entails. *Please tell me about what you think will happen while you are in hospital* can elicit a revealing account of expectations, and sometimes information about what the patient thinks that nurses, doctors and others do.

Each of the remaining three sorts of person-centred care work builds upon anticipating care requirements (evidence utilisation) and narrative analysis, and each depends on what sort of partnership can be established with the patient.

- Unless we understand what patients think might constitute a risk (real or imagined) we cannot counter worries and agree on a confident way forward. We learn about their perceptions through the narrative analysis work.
- We cannot agree on how best to work with the patient unless we understand what role they think patients play. In some care situations patients refuse to partner nurses in care. Instead they accept the minimum treatment necessary to correct a deficit and hope that further introspection and adaptation is unnecessary.
- We can only evaluate the success of care with the patient if we agree criteria for what counts as success. Through listening attentively to the patient narrative we ascertain what they hope for, that which would seem successful to them.

Patients may be extremely inquisitive, proactive and interested partners, in many ways the ideal patient of person-centred care. But they may equally be passive, expecting that treatment and care will happen to them. They may insist that they trust the healthcare staff and wish to simply respond to the instructions of doctors and nurses. Other patients are suspicious, perhaps even aggressive or untruthful, so the nurse has to regularly review their impressions in order to assess what is possible in terms of a care partnership.

As you have worked through the patient case studies you may have been struck by the different patient and lay carer responses when nurses have invited them to become involved in care planning. If the patient suffers from depression, it might be extremely difficult for them to share their feelings in a care partnership. Motivation is itself problematic when each day seems such a challenge. If the lay carer is extremely anxious, then they might make demands on the nurse, some of which contradict what they try to do in supporting the patient. The nurse has to demonstrate respect to the carer, engaging them in care thinking, so that they understand what might prove therapeutic. If a child suffers from diabetes mellitus, or is dying, it might be harder for the parent to contain their anxieties, to make sense of what they can do to help, so partnership with the nurse might have to involve a three-way interaction.

To implement person-centred care involves strategy, engaging in different work at different stages of care. Good work done at the start of the care relationship may establish a good working relationship later, or at least mitigate some of the doubts and suspicions that the patient has brought to healthcare. The extent to which person-centred care is successful depends on approach and skills (evidence use and narrative listening) but it depends too on patient expectations of partnership and the different patient activity that might be required there (e.g., learning, becoming more self-motivated, exploring beliefs and feelings). Through their partnerships with patients, nurses have a vital role in facilitating change.

Activity 9.1 Reflecting

Looking back over the case studies that you have read, would you agree that the recurring three themes are using evidence to best effect, understanding the patient/lay carer narrative and managing a care partnership?

Make a note of which of these, in your experience, might seem the most exciting and the most difficult to arrange. So, for example, when you take up your new post in a clinical specialism, how interesting/feasible will it seem to get to know evidence about those patients really well? What in your experience of talking with patients makes it either easy or difficult to elicit their experience of illness or care? Do you think that patients are clear about their role in healthcare and what a partnership with the nurse might entail?

As this activity is based on your own reflection, no sample answer is provided at the end of the chapter.

What can or should be expected of care partnership?

Your answer regarding the three sorts of future work in Activity 9.1 may well have depended on things such as how confident you feel locating and reading research papers or interviewing patients. But I suspect that the greatest challenge that most readers will have anticipated relates to the sort of care partnerships that nurses can develop with patients. Your clinical experience placements are likely to have acquainted you with just how diverse, delightful, confusing and sometimes awkward patients can seem. An hour or two watching a TV healthcare soap opera rapidly reminds us that many of the care challenges that we face are not just to do with clinical risks and challenges but with relating to people. Patients come to healthcare with a host of unexpressed expectations and some new expectations are discovered while developing care relationships. Patients come to care with widely varying abilities to express their expectations. Some patients may feel damaged by unsuccessful care relationships in the past.

Given the importance of care partnering to the success of person-centred care in the future, it is important to ascertain why such problems arise. Beyond the observation that people are different and we cannot possibly always anticipate what their expectations of healthcare might be, one major challenge that confronts us in the future relates to patient role. Patients might not know what their role should be or, conversely, they may try to dictate the care relationship, allocating the nurse an instruction-taking role. A patient might be an aggressive consumer, requiring the nurse to follow their requirements, sometimes with little regard to clinical risks. Partnership can sometimes become political, even ideological, in nature.

Whether or not individual patients seem collaborative, awkward, or difficult, there are systemic problems that have contributed to this issue.

In 2014 NHS England published its five-year plan for the future of English healthcare (*Five Year Forward View*). It emphasised the challenge of arranging healthcare in the face of growing demands, an ageing population and the advances afforded by technology and medicine. When demands are many and resources are few, choices have to be made. It is in the arranging of choices, the managing of resources and the attending to clients of the service that NHS England has thought again.

Reflecting on the past NHS, the prospectus (p9) observes:

> *Sometimes the health service has been prone to operating a 'factory' model of care and repair, with limited engagement with the wider community, a short-sighted approach to partnerships, and under-developed advocacy and action on the broader influencers of health and wellbeing.*

Put simply, the document observes that the NHS has become the victim of its own success and that the early aspirations to provide a cradle-to-grave system, one rescuing patients, has tended to encourage greater and greater demands by the public. Instead of helping to equip the public to take preventative action, there has been an emphasis on reactive treatment and care, leaving the weight of responsibility upon healthcare services and professionals. This problem is reaching a crisis point where it is increasingly difficult for nurses and others to practice with confidence.

NHS England acknowledge that failures in public and preventative health continue to fuel pressures within the treatment and support services of the NHS.

In the *Five Year Forward View* (NHS England, 2014) three major objectives were identified, those that were described as ongoing in the progress report published in 2017 (NHS England, 2017).

1. To radically upgrade the preventative and public health services (helping to stem the pressures on corrective healthcare).
2. To enable patients to secure far greater control of their own care.
3. To break down barriers in how care was delivered.

In 2018 Health Education England (Willis) published a document (*Raising the Bar: Shape of Caring*) on how nursing should facilitate the goals of the *Five Year Forward View*. This envisaged a much more wide-ranging leadership role for nurses. Significantly, it recommended that student nurses would spend two years of their learning on 'whole person care training', an elective year in a specialist training, followed by one year under preceptorship. The report recommends that there should be much greater involvement of patients and lay carers in the education of nurses.

What is clear within this collection of documents is that there is encouragement to innovate locally and to find better ways to engage patients, lay carers and other agencies (social as well as healthcare) as part of a more seamless and nimble patient support. As the pressures grow upon the NHS, there is an urgent need to reconceive of care. The limited resource of time, staff, equipment and facilities will have to work better. But there would also need to be much more emphasis on partnership.

What government planning fails to specify, however, are expectations of individual members of the public as regards the maintenance of health (preventing illness or injury) and then, within bounds of individual patient financial and other resources, what patients are expected to do when partnering healthcare professionals in care. This uncertainty about individual responsibility is problematic because it leaves nurses with little indication of what they can reasonably expect patients to do. While nursing supports care partnership, there is little indication of what patient responsibility exists or entails. In no other form of partnership does a professional have quite such an unstructured arrangement to deal with.

In such contexts, it is not surprising that care partnership can prove problematic for patients and for nurses. The nurse must at once use his or her expertise to recommend, and yet work sensitively with, the patient as they come to terms with their new circumstances. Without clearer cultural, political or social norms guidance on looking after oneself, on remaining well, the nurse might find that the patient selects from any number of roles of their own choosing, including those that make partnership very difficult indeed.

The lack of government guidance is perhaps no less confusing and perplexing for the public. If we start with health, members of the public are confronted with rapidly changing science updates on risks associated with such things as diet, weight management, exercise, stress at work and environment hazards. Sometimes the research guidance conflicts, for instance on safe levels of alcohol consumption or the merits and demerits of a modest intake of alcohol. Science is not necessarily guiding the public on how best to live and that can mean that patients become more cautious about trusting the advice of healthcare professionals.

While young people may have been taught about such things as personal hygiene, the value of a balanced diet, how to avoid sexually transmitted disease and the benefits of vaccinations, there has not been a coherent syllabus within public education on health maintenance. Instead, teaching has centred on countering particular risks. This casts the individual as someone who reacts to a problem, rather than one who develops a lifestyle that acknowledges significant responsibility for health maintenance and that accepts the necessity to accept and manage risks.

If individuals then enter the healthcare system ill-prepared to regulate their own health, manage challenges, seize opportunities, they are then poorly positioned when nurses and doctors set challenges associated with managing an illness, working with medication or coping with the long-term uncertainty of a threat such as cancer.

The nurse, in effect, has to teach the patient to confront new responsibilities and in a context where the public may think of healthcare as rescue and resolution. The nurse may have to challenge lifestyle, to question patient assumptions, and recommend practices that limit clinical risks.

Despite these challenges, there remain some interesting possibilities that nurses could explore. Each of those summarised below have the potential to facilitate person-centred care in the future.

Taking the professional lead on public health education

While many professionals are engaged in public health education, it is arguable that nurses are well placed to lead on promoting health, sustaining a sense of well-being and taking personal responsibility for managing a range of risks that exist as part of life. This has to be achieved without promoting a 'nanny state'. In order to make adult and independent decisions, human beings need to understand the merits, challenges, possibilities and risks of different lifestyle choices. Nurses are intimately aware of the consequences of poor health decisions, and they help manage the experience of threat, loss and recovery when illness, disability or injury intervenes. Nurses have an expressed interest in how patients reason risk, how they conceive of coping and loss, and they are practised, through analysis of patient narratives, in helping individuals to think about change in more accessible terms. While scientists report findings and add to the growing evidence that describes risks and benefits, nurses are engaged in helping others to weigh up evidence. Nurses advise people in the context of their life circumstances, such as, for example, about diet when budgets are limited.

There is then a case for nursing as a profession to spend more time and effort in lifestyle teaching. Nurses might, for example, teach members of the public how to anticipate and manage ageing, how to compensate for limits in mobility. Risk is not inherently bad (humans thrive on stimuli) and we cannot entirely remove risk from life. However, analysing the likelihood of harm occurring and its significance if it does can help people make better lifestyle choices. Health and illness are a continuum. Members of the public spend a great deal of time dealing with developing health deficits long before they bring these to the attention of the healthcare services. Nurses have potential to make a difference in public education. Nurses are also accustomed to helping individuals think about what they could do, as well as recommending what they should do. One patient once described this to me as 'they know' teaching. The advice to re-evaluate risks was accepted because the nurse helped the individual to find acceptable ways to change.

Contracting realistic and explicit care plans

The second promising measure is to contract care objectives more honestly with patients. Patients may come to care negotiation with very different expectations but it is possible to help a patient realise what more might be achieved if shared responsibilities for care are embraced. One nurse put it this way [I paraphrase]:

Realistically I cannot provide my patient with perfect care. Some less well-resourced or infirm patients I have to give more of my time to. But for the others, I sometimes describe what can be achieved in terms of three levels.

The first is that achieved if the patient is passive and leaves me to address as many of their care needs in the time and resources available. Of course that care has to be considerate and supportive, but it is necessarily finite.

The second level of care relates to that which might be achieved if the patient and I work in partnership. For example, if he persists with some physiotherapy beyond the sessions that I teach. What might be achieved then is greater, perhaps in terms of speed of recovery or the range of movements secured. One patient said to me, 'being a patient is a job of work, isn't it?' and he was right.

The third level of outcome, the best, is where the patient learns to do new things, to think of themselves in new ways and goes on changing after he or she has left my care. Then the achievements possible are significantly improved.

So when I sit down with a patient I sometimes ask, 'how much do you want to achieve?' If I didn't take that approach, then it would be hard to keep going as a nurse.

Finding new ways to help patients to learn

As you may have realised in this book, much of successful healthcare is closely related to the patient's ability and willingness to learn. The more that the patient understands and commands as regards self-care, the greater their freedom to live in personally meaningful ways. If restorative care cannot entirely cure the patient, absolving them of problem-solving requirements, learning to cope and then change becomes vital. Sometimes the learning work involves confrontation. A patient may assume that the service corrects all difficulties. It is then necessary, politely, to explain the merits of learning self-care abilities, those that facilitate independence. Explaining what learning will enable the patient to do (opportunity motivating) is likely to be more successful than stating that such learning will save the NHS x amount of money (moral motivating). The goal is to present learning as a win–win opportunity. It's in this area that the nurse has a chance to work with NHS England (2014) and Health Education England (Willis) (2018) objectives to empower patients. The nurse persuades the patient and lay carers of the merits of learning. Whether learning is best done collectively or individually is something you explored in the case studies of this book. However, there remains scope to enquire and innovate further. For example, it is worth examining just how powerful patient role-modelling might be in the teaching of others. If a respected patient can be helped to better articulate their successful coping, does that help sustain the efforts of patients who come after them?

Opening leadership discussions with others

Health Education England (Willis) (2018) are a little coy about leadership and change within the NHS, referring briefly to the merits of *collective leadership*. There is, however, scope for local teams to work rather more honestly in this area. Once acute care and treatment have been completed, there is considerable scope for nurses to lead as the key worker in support of groups of patients. This is an area, in rehabilitation and chronic care, where well-educated person-centred nurses can excel. If nurses research to better effect, using evidence well, and maximise their understanding of narratives, there is no reason why nurses might not create a post-acute care exemplary service, that which is clearly effective, efficient and person-centred. For this to work, however, frank discussions need to take place with regard to the system for conferring, referring and problem-solving patient caseloads. Just as person-centred care clearly relies on the collective resources of the service, so it requires clear responsibility for who liaises with the patient and family on care.

Activity 9.2   Enquiring

The above arguments about the need to clarify public and patient responsibilities regarding health and illness resolution are quite frank, aren't they? They suggest a shift in the approach of the nurse, one that requires more expectation of others in partnership. Explore now with clinicians that you know whether they agree with the need to gradually redefine partnership working. What do they think is necessary to enable the nurse to help customise care more sensitively, effectively and efficiently?

As this activity is based on your own reflection, no sample answer is provided at the end of the chapter.

What about person-centred care might best sustain your satisfaction in care delivery?

In the final section of the chapter I want to refer to four papers that span nearly 20 years of nursing. What I think is remarkable about them is that, collectively, they demonstrate the lack of progress made as regards understanding and nurturing the motivation of nurses. Correcting this is important, not just to the furtherance of person-centred care but in sustaining nursing more generally. We know that today there is a shortage of nurses, that many in practice are already in their 50s and 60s, and that it takes time to recruit and educate replacements when health services are so evidently under pressure (Kwok et al., 2016). We need to enthuse nurse learners, to sustain registered nurse practitioners and to keep colleagues happier in practice despite the stress of work over time.

The first paper reports a small-sample qualitative data study by Jenny Spouse (2000). Spouse interviewed five student nurses to understand their aspirations in nursing. Each of the nurses were motivated slightly differently, but I think that the emergent themes might seem remarkably familiar to you. One of the respondents (Ruth) dealt with the sharp contrasts between what she hoped to deliver as care and what the environment allowed. This was expressed in terms of the difference between a 'loving attitude' and reality. A second student (Nicola) emphasised the importance of listening to patients and (in some sense) being with them. Rebecca, a student who finally left her studies, admitted that she had no preconceived notion of what nursing would be like. She discovered, however, that nurses, managers and the public had widely differing expectations of the nurse's role.

Today, I suspect that the ambiguities remain. Person-centred care remains a project designed to allow nurses to feel compassionate as well as to deliver individualised care. That which motivates nurses strongly is the wish to see others not only improve in material health terms but with regard to how they feel about their circumstances.

This emphasis on compassion as something that motivates nurses was reported again in a larger study of 126 nurses by Burtson and Stichler (2010). In the analysis of what constituted nursing care for these respondents, the opportunity to express compassion accounted for nearly a third of all answers received. While nurses did things, demonstrated skills and shared knowledge, the facility to signal their compassion and to see that their work made a difference remained vitally important. Compassion, however, remained a two-edged sword. Just as compassion was a key motivator for nurses so it could also be a source of burn-out. What was vital in sustaining nurses was the due balance of compassion-expression opportunity. Nurses needed to be able to express compassion, but not to have circumstances so ambiguously arranged that they couldn't manage its emotional demands.

Just how taxing this is was described by Shea (2015) writing about nurse practitioners. Such senior clinicians might be expected to have greater outlet for their professional aspirations, but the themes described remained remarkably similar. The 15 nurses felt fuelled when care arrangements were sufficiently in their control to seem coherent with professional values, including the expression of compassion. But care was extremely frustrating when it seemed compromised because they could not offer adequate resource themselves or negotiate similar from elsewhere.

Writing about nurse retention from a management perspective, Kwok et al. (2016) noted that keeping older nurses in Canadian posts was firmly about practical support measures, such as flexible shift work, but it was also about the experience of caring. To sustain care motivation, to manage the changes in systems and technologies, it was important to provide nurses with mentor support, so that they could be helped to review, redefine and remain excited about their role.

It would be easy to conclude, from papers such as those described above, that the system is letting nursing down. We are less able to deliver person-centred care because systems, resources and public expectations have seen nursing in quite ambiguous and sometimes conflicting ways. Nurses are vocational people who care, we are technicians and skilled practitioners, we counsel, teach and lead. I think that there is much truth in such arguments, but I venture, too, that we do ourselves a disservice if we think that person-centred care is brought about entirely through a fix to the system. While, as I indicate above, there does need to be a review of care partner assumptions, better education of the public and a review of how care is led, I also think that there are opportunities for us to use what motivates us best to secure pleasure from care-giving. That which sustains a nurse and keeps them working creatively within the service may be about targeting some reflection that connects practitioner and patient satisfaction.

I believe that there are four things that provide prompt and important pleasure in delivering care. None of these is solely determined by the service or the healthcare system that we work within. They are all strongly associated with how we relate to patients, moment by moment.

Discovering that we understand the patient better than expected

One of the benefits of conducting and using patient experience research of the kind described in this book is that we have the opportunity to try out explanations of need, recognition of concern, with the next patients that we meet. There evolves a recurring, empathetic experiment in which the nurse offers thoughts, insights, reflections from their store of evidence and monitors patient response. Asking patients *what do you think?* or *is it like that for you?* can be extremely rewarding. Imagining, through evidence, how a situation might seem to a patient is a powerful expression of compassion. *I care enough about you to have explored what often causes concern.* When that patient then confirms something as insightful, helpful, caring, kind, the nurse secures a powerful feedback. It is not that nurses simply need a 'fix' of compassion recognition, it is that such feedback sustains and modifies their approach to care over the longer term. The nurse who secures such high-quality feedback from patients and lay carers is motivated to go on learning through practice. Work seems less a job and more a personal opportunity. It becomes a means to be a nurse as well as to work as one.

Discovering an admiration for the patient and what they do

People are wonderfully different. While we might catalogue illnesses in terms of signs, symptoms, aetiology and prognosis, we cannot nor should we catalogue people in that way. People define their situation in different ways and they use different coping strategies to manage what they are confronted with. We only start to understand and to appreciate those insights into people and their way of living when we hear and reflect on the narratives that they share. The patient (if we will permit them) tells us a story of their lot. They convey their efforts to counter the problems that have arisen. We materially need to understand this if we are to suggest better ways to cope and resources that might seem especially useful to them.

But there is a personal and altruistic reason to enquire into the narratives that the patient shares as well. This is the search for admiration and respect. Professionalism (managing distance with the patient) should not exclude humanity. It seems to me that it is much easier to commit to nursing, to come back eager to care over time, when I have found a respect and an admiration for the patient and their relatives. We might not be able to change all of their circumstances, but we can keep on engaging, assuring and sustaining the patient the more we respect what they do.

Without hearing and finding things to admire in the narratives shared by those we care for, the person is at risk of remaining just a patient. It is necessary to search for things to acknowledge in their own self-care. *I'd never thought of that, but it works, you seem so much less anxious thinking about things in that way.* Mutual respect, and even admiration, sustains caring relationships. We create opportunities for the relationship formed to be seen in incrementally better terms.

Discovering that we have modest tools to help the patient

I wonder how grand you thought the interventions are in the case study chapters of this book? Were they especially technological, profound and resource-rich? I suspect that you might answer no. What the nurse and colleagues have done, in most circumstances, has been to talk differently, to refer the patient or relatives to really good sources of assistance or to modestly adjust the environment in which the patient encounters illness and treatment. This, as well as compassion, defines nursing. Whatever else we do, that which defines our contribution is how we relate to patients and help them find ways forward. The person-centred contributions of the nurse can be both discrete and powerful. That which the patient remembers, that which they might yet act upon to improve their health, may be the expression of the nurse's kindness.

When I have pressed patients to explain what they mean when they say that a nurse was 'kind' they have found it hard to explain matters. There is a sense in which the nurse attends to the patient, the way that they listen and confirm their hearing of that which has been said. But I think that 'kind' is usually code for 'helpful' as well. Kind nurses, remembered, valued and attitude-influential nurses, have been those that have suggested ways in which problems might be understood and choices made. The patient might accept one or more of the suggestions, but what is sometimes just as important is that the nurse has alerted them to possibilities.

It's worth dwelling on this, the pleasure of seeing a patient better-equipped. The patient might not select the option we might have chosen, but then we are not the patient and our resources and circumstances are different. It is unhelpful to indict ourselves if they do not follow our recommendation. Healthcare is an advisory matter, with benefits and risks reviewed. The better and often the more pleasurable reflection concerns a review of whether we enabled them to clarify what seemed possible for them. If we persist in seeing care as a zero sum game, where there is only satisfaction in persuading a patient to a quite specific course of action, it is likely to seem harder sustaining ourselves in practice.

Discovering that patients appreciate what we do (personally)

I wonder if we always hear the thank yous accurately. I wonder if we allow those thank yous to sustain us in our efforts to deliver more person-centred care. It can be difficult to dwell on a thank you expressed. For one thing, it seems egoistic and unprofessional. We are accustomed to dismissing our efforts. Either care is vocational/instinctive, or else 'it's what we're paid to do'. I think that neither of these responses are sufficient. They close down the feedback on to next good practice. We learn little from a thank you, just that we have done a good job, or else been 'nice'.

What marks out receiving thank yous to better personal satisfaction and professional effect is understanding how or why the care delivered was especially appreciated. Delivering the person-centred care of the future will depend upon belief. It will depend on believing that working in particular ways are recognised as valuable. If nurses are not to simply act as generic care workers, then it is important that they articulate, from patient and relative feedback, just how they have improved the experience of healthcare services. No matter how much a theorist, philosopher or textbook writer suggests what person-centred care is, matters are only improved and gains protected when we find ways of helping patients articulate their appreciation as well as their criticism. I wonder if that sounds like a point about service? Well, it is, but it is also about your pleasure as well. That which works, which is recognised, which you enjoy doing, you will go on doing more of for the rest of your career.

Chapter summary

I have reached the end of this glimpse forward into the future and indeed of the book as a whole.

This book has set out to try and show how person-centred care can be exemplified in daily practice. It has illustrated the often simple and discrete measures that seem to make a difference for patients. It is sometimes the relatively subtle, the interpersonal measures that nurses use that register with patients as person-centred and as especially professional and kind.

This chapter makes a number of speculative points about the future of person-centred care.

(Continued)

(Continued)

- Care in the future is likely to be substantially influenced by the ways in which healthcare is conceived and arranged. Initiatives to involve patients more in care design and planning are encouraging, but the success of person-centred care will depend on much else done within healthcare services, for instance that taught to the public about health and wellbeing.
- Because person-centred care is so intimately related to the notion of partnership, it is vital that the role of the patient as a co-designer of care is clarified. If patients are to be partners then their rights and responsibilities need to be clarified.
- Strategic use can and should be made of qualitative research evidence on the experience of patients, their response to illness and the ways in which they relate to healthcare professionals. The more the nurse can anticipate the more wise they may seem to subsequent patients.
- Nurses need to press on with their study of patient and relative narratives for it is through these that we better understand patient need, motivation and facility as a partner in care.
- The development and sustaining of nurses over a career in nursing needs to return afresh to what motivates nurses. In many instances this is the opportunity to express not only their expertise but their compassion as well.

Further reading

I want to finish by commending three books to you, all of which might prove useful in association with previous chapters as much as with this one. No recommended websites are offered this time, as I believe contemplation of texts such as these has greater merit.

Plummer, D (2010) *Helping Children to Cope with Change, Stress and Anxiety.* London: Jessica Kingsley Publishing.

I start with a very practical guide, largely aimed at parents and designed to help them steer children through the transitions linked to growing up. I think that helping others through change is what person-centred care often focusses upon so it is valuable to contemplate that.

Hasson, G (2018) *Kindness.* Chichester: Wiley and Sons (Capstone).

Hasson's book is a very practical examination of kindness, and if you sometimes worry that this has been left out of nursing care then this book will encourage and reassure you. There are many ways to express kindness.

Walker, L (2009) *Persuasion in Clinical Practice: Helping People Make Changes.* Oxford: Radcliffe Publishing.

Walker's primary audience is doctors but it is refreshing and encouraging to find a text such as this on the healthcare learning agenda. It's very tempting for clinicians to simply tell patients what they need to take, what they need to do. Walker, however, is keenly aware that patients are in varying states of readiness to listen to clinicians' recommendations.

Glossary of key terms

clinical need   That need associated with the management of risks to the patient and the effective and efficient use of treatment (see also **felt need**).

consumer-led care   Care that responds to the needs of groups of patients working together or individually to meet requirements associated with particular illnesses or treatment-related needs. While the individual patient as a consumer may research their requirements, they may also be represented by pressure groups working in their sectional interests.

discourse   A positional statement or series of arguments that express our values or our understanding of events. So, within nursing, there is a discourse about what person-centred care should look like. In palliative care there is a discourse associated with end of life care. Discourses compete and clash within healthcare making it harder for us to know how best to proceed. To support a discourse we need to understand the underpinning premises and the values and beliefs that are attached.

empowering/empowerment   Enabling patients to take increasing control and responsibility regarding their illness and associated needs. It is furthered by sharing information, building confidence and enabling the patient to learn.

expert patient   A patient who has become knowledgeable and skilful as regards a well-understood illness and the associated treatment and support requirements. Expert patients are capable of guiding and teaching others (including healthcare staff) regarding their needs.

felt need   The need experienced and sometimes expressed by patients and lay carers. Felt need tends to relate to patients dealing with illness in the context of their own lives. It is a contextual, perceptual and aspirational need. Felt need does not necessarily take into account the competing needs of other patients or the finite resources of a service. A felt need might be either judicious (therapeutic) or injudicious (something that could cause harm).

holism   The belief that the individual is best understood as the sum of many parts; their physical, psychological, spiritual and social dimensions. Holism drove much of nursing development in the second half of the twentieth century, although opportunities to express care in each dimension were often limited.

managerialism   A broad and often pejorative term used to describe changes within healthcare services designed to ensure that services work more efficiently and effectively. The introduction of managers was seen by some healthcare professionals as an implicit criticism of the control that they exercised and the way in which practitioners managed finite resources.

metacognition   Understanding ourselves and how we act. The nurse who is metacognitive understands his or her role and the way in which care philosophy contributes to that role.

motivation   That which sustains individuals in their efforts and that which makes activities meaningful. Understanding motivation is important if patients are to learn well and to maintain self care in adverse circumstances (see Chapter 7). There are different ways of describing motivation. It may be driven by a search for rewards, or by an increasing sense of purpose linked to meaningful activities that help confirm a satisfying identity.

narrative   A story or explanation embedded within a series of words; the dialogues shared with others. The narrative may convey how we see ourselves, how we cope with illness, or (as a nurse or lay carer) how we try to care. Narratives may be hidden. Sometimes the nurse has to check carefully what patients are in fact conveying in their narrative.

patient role   That which the person is expected to do while they are receiving treatment and care through health services. Historically, the patient role was well defined in terms of responsibilities and rights (Parsons, 1951) but, in modern times, the role has been reconceived of in negotiating terms. At one extreme the patient acts as a consumer, a critical appraiser of service. At another extreme the patient is a co-care companion, sharing in the identification and the solving of problems.

person-centred care (pragmatic)   Care that centres on the person within a healthcare system that sets significant limits on resources, and which serves the many as well as the individual. Pragmatic person-centred care elucidates role responsibilities for the nurse and the patient, acknowledging the expertise that the nurse brings to bear in the service of the patient (see the full definition on pp20–1, Chapter 1).

personhood   That which distinguishes us as whole and different from others. The person is defined by their abilities, and aptitudes, by their attitudes and values and through the relationships that they share with others. Illness and treatment may undermine personhood through its impact on the body and on our sense of control over daily living.

philosophical person-centred care   Care that centres on the needs, requirements and hopes of the person and, beyond that, is simply associated with their role as a patient. Person-centred care in its philosophical sense also expresses the aspirations of nursing as a profession and idealised care relationships (see Chapter 1).

rapport   A mutual state of respect and understanding, in which each understands and appreciates the contribution of the other.

therapeutic relationship   That which describes how the nurse and patient relate to one another in ways that achieve beneficial ends. To be therapeutic the nurse musters communication and clinical skills and makes selective use of evidence to guide the patient. The relationship extends to become a culture where a wide range of staff and services are marshalled so as to advance the needs of the individual patient.

References

Abell, B, Glasziou, P, Briffa, T and Hoffman, T (2015) Exercise training characteristics in cardiac rehabilitation programmes: a cross sectional survey of Australian practice. *Open Heart*, doi: 10.1136/openhrt-2015-00374

Abotalebidariasari, G, Memarian, R, Vanaki, Z et al. (2016) Self care motivation among patients with heart failure: a qualitative study based on Orem's theory. *Research and Theory for Nursing Practice*, *30* (4): 320–32.

Adams, K, Cimino, J and Arnold, R et al. (2012) Why should I talk about emotion? Communication patterns associated with physician discussion of patient expressions of negative emotion in hospital admission encounters. *Patient Education and Counselling*, *89* (1): 44–50.

Adams, N and Grieder, D (2013) *Treatment Planning for Person-Centred Care: Shared Decision Making for Whole Health* (2nd edition). Edinburgh: Elsevier Science.

Alsen, P and Eriksson, M (2016) Illness perceptions of fatigue and the association with sense of coherence and stress in patients one year after myocardial infarction. *Journal of Clinical Nursing*, *25*: 526–33.

Alshmemri, M, Shahwan-Akl, L and Maude, P (2017) Herzberg's Two-Factor Theory. *Life Science Journal*, *14* (5): 12–16.

American Cancer Society (2018) *Treatment of Colon Cancer by Stage*. Available online at: www.cancer.org/colon-rectal-cancer/treating/by-stage-colon.html

Anderson, C and Tapesh, R (2013) Patient experiences of taking antidepressants for depression: a secondary qualitative analysis. *Research in Social and Administrative Pharmacy*, *9* (6): 884–902.

Anderson, L, Oldridge, N, Thompson, D et al. (2016) Exercise-based cardiac rehabilitation for coronary heart disease. *Journal of American College of Cardiology*, *67* (1): 1–12.

Anuradha, S (2015) Effect of a structured teaching programme on prevention of hypoglycaemia among diabetic patients. *International Journal of Nursing Education*, *7* (4), 47–52.

Avery, A, Whitehead, K and Halliday, V (2016) *How to Facilitate Lifestyle Change: Applying Group Education in Healthcare*. Chichester: Wiley Blackwell.

Barclay, S, Frogatt, K, Crang, C et al. (2014) Living in uncertain times: trajectories to death in residential care homes. *The British Journal of General Practice*, *64* (626): e576–e583.

Bartol, T (2014) Integrating behavioral health: building a relationship of hope. *The Nurse Practitioner*, *39* (12): 10–12.

Baruch, G (1981) Moral tales: parents' stories of encounters with health professionals. *Sociology of Health and Illness, 3* (3): 275–95.

Bennett, E, English, M, Rennoldson, M et al. (2013) Predicting parenting stress in care givers of children with brain tumours. *Psycho-Oncology, 22* (3): 629–36.

Bergh, A, Karlsson, J, Persson, E et al. (2012) Registered nurses' perceptions of conditions for patient education: focusing on organizational, environmental and professional cooperation aspects. *Journal of Nursing Management, 20*: 758–70.

Bewtra, M, Kilambi, V, Fairchild, A et al. (2014) Patient preferences for surgical versus medical therapy for ulcerative colitis. *Inflammatory Bowel Diseases, 20* (1): 103–14.

Bigi, S (2014) Key concepts of effective collaborative goal setting in the chronic care encounter. *Communication and Medicine, 11* (2): 103–15.

Blair, J, Anthony, T, Gunther, I et al. (2017) A protocol for the preparation of patients for theatre and recovery. *Learning Disability Practice, 20* (2): 22–6.

Bluebond-Langner, M (1978) *The Private Worlds of Dying Children*. Princeton, NJ: Princeton University Press.

Borreani, C, Giordano, A, Falautano, M et al. (2014) Experience of an information aid for newly diagnosed multiple sclerosis patients: a qualitative study of the SIMS-Trial. *Health Expectations, 17* (1): 36–48.

Brand, J, Kopke, S, Kasper, J et al. (2014) Magnetic resonance imaging in multiple sclerosis: patients' experiences, information interests and responses to an education plan. *PLOS One, 9* (11): e113252.

Brittan, N, Moore, L, Lydhal, D et al. (2016) Elaboration of the Gothenburg model of person-centred care. *Health Expectations, 20*: 407–18.

Brooker, C and Waugh, A (2013) *Foundations of Nursing Practice: Fundamentals of Holistic Care* (2nd edition). Edinburgh: Mosby/Elsevier.

Brown, P, Morello-Frosch, R and Zavostocki, S (2011) *Contested Illnesses: Citizens, Science and Health Social Movements*. Berkeley, CA: University of California Press.

Brown, R, Barbour, P and Martin, D (2015) *The Mental Capacity Act 2005: A Guide For Practice* (3rd edition). London: SAGE/Learning Matters.

Browning, S and Waite, R (2010) The gift of listening: JUST listening strategies. *Nursing Forum, 45* (3): 150–8.

Burtson, P and Stichler, J (2010) Nursing work environment and nurse caring relationship among motivational factors. *Journal of Advanced Nursing, 66* (8): 1819–31.

Butts, J and Rich, K (2014) *Philosophies and Theories for Advanced Nursing Practice* (2nd edition). Burlington, MA: Jones and Bartlett.

Calnan, M (2010) Consumerism and the provision of healthcare. *British Journal of Healthcare Management, 16* (1): 37–9.

Campbell, H (2014) *Nursing and Health Palliative Care Survival Guide*. Abingdon: Routledge.

Carmichael, M and Bridge, P (2017) Expert patient perspectives on radiotherapy: a phenomenological comparison. *Journal of Radiotherapy in Practice, 16* (2): 207–14.

Ceccarini, M, Manzoni, G and Castelnouvo, G (2014) Assessing depression in cardiac patients: what measures should be considered? *Depression Research and Treatment*, Epub 6 February: 1–17.

Clark, R, Conway, A, Poulson, V et al. (2015) Alternative models of cardiac rehabilitation: a systematic review. *European Journal of Preventative Cardiology, 22* (1): 35–74.

Codling, M (2015) Helping service users to take control of their health. *Learning Disability Practice, 18* (3): doi: 10.7748/ldp.18.3.26.e1612

Conklin, L and Strunk, D (2015) A session-to-session examination of homework engagement in cognitive therapy for depression: do patients experience immediate benefits? *Behavioural Research and Therapy, 72*: 56–62.

Cope, V, Jones, B and Hendricks, J (2015) Resilience as resistance to the new managerialism: portraits that reframe nursing through quotes from the field. *Journal of Nursing Management, 24* (1): 115–22.

Counselling Directory (2018) *Mental Health Facts and Figures*. Available online at: www.counselling-directory-org.uk/stats.html

Coventry, L, Schalkwyk, J, Thompson, P et al. (2017) Myocardial infarction patient decision delay and help-seeking behavior: a thematic analysis. *Journal of Clinical Nursing, 26* (13–14): 1993–2005.

Cowie, H (2012) *From Birth to Sixteen Years: Children's Health, Social, Emotional and Cognitive Development*. Abingdon: Routledge.

Davies, F, Edwards, A, Brain, K et al. (2015) 'You are just left to get on with it': qualitative study of patient and carer experiences of the transition to secondary progressive multiple sclerosis. *BMJ Open, 5* (7): doi: 10.1136/bmjopen-2015-007674

Dennison, L, Moss-Morris, R, Yardley, L et al. (2013) Change and processes of change within interventions to promote adjustment to multiple sclerosis: learning from patient experiences. *Psychology and Health, 28* (9): 973–92.

Department of Health (1989a) *Working for Patients* (White Paper). London: HM Govt, Department of Health.

Department of Health (1989b) *Caring for People: Community Care in the Next Decade and Beyond* (White Paper). London: HM Govt, Department of Health.

Desmond Project (2018) *Developing Quality Structured Education in Diabetes*. Available online at: www.desmond.project.org.uk

Doblyte, S and Jimenez-Mejias, E (2017) Understanding help-seeking behavior in depression: a qualitative synthesis of patients' experiences. *Qualitative Health Research, 27* (1): 100–13.

Doherty, M and Thompson, H (2014) Enhancing person-centred care through the development of the therapeutic relationship. *British Journal of Community Nursing, 19* (10): 504–7.

Dozeman, E, Van Marwijk, H, Van Schaik, D et al. (2012) Contradictory effects for prevention of depression and anxiety in residents in homes for the elderly: a pragmatic randomized controlled trial. *International Psychogeriatrics, 24* (8): 1242–51.

Drozd, M and Clinch, C (2016) The experiences of orthopaedic and trauma nurses who have cared for adults with a learning disability. *International Journal of Orthopaedic and Trauma Nursing, 22*: 13–23.

Dunpath, T, Chetty, V and Van der Reyden, D (2015) The experience of acute burns of the hand: patient perspectives. *Disability and Rehabilitation, 37* (10): 892.

Elwyn, G, Edwards, A and Thompson, A (2016) *Shared Decision Making in Healthcare: Achieving Evidence-Based Patient Choice.* Oxford: Oxford University Press.

Feldman, R, Dunner, D, Muller, J et al. (2013) Medicare patient experience with vagus nerve stimulation for treatment resistant depression. *Journal of Medical Economics, 16* (1): 62–74.

Figueiras, M, Maroco, J, Monteiro, R et al. (2017) Randomized controlled trial of an intervention to change cardiac misconceptions in myocardial infarction patients. *Psychology, Health and Medicine, 22* (3): 255–65.

Forman, D (2016) Cardiac rehabilitation: the mandate grows. *Mayo Clinic Proceedings, 91* (2): 125–8.

Frank, L, Matza, L, Handon, J et al. (2007) The patient experience of depression and remission: focus group results. *Journal of Nervous and Mental Disease, 195* (8): 647–54.

Furingsten, L, Sjogren, R and Forsner, M (2015) Ethical challenges when caring for dying children. *Nursing Ethics, 22* (2): 176–87.

Gabe, J and Calnan, M (2009) *The New Sociology of the Health Service.* Abingdon: Routledge.

Gabrielsson, S, Savenstedt, S and Zingmark, K (2014) Person-centred care: clarifying the concept in the context of inpatient psychiatry. *Scandinavian Journal of Caring Sciences, 29*: 555–62.

Ghafari, S, Fellahi-Khoshknab, M, Nourozi, K et al. (2015) Patients' experiences of adapting to multiple sclerosis: a qualitative study. *Contemporary Nurse, 50* (1): 36–49.

Ghisi, G, Grace, S, Thomas, S and Oh, P (2015) Behavioral determinants among cardiac rehabilitation patients receiving educational interventions: an application of the health action process approach. *Patient Education and Counselling, 98* (5): 612–21.

Ginicola, M, Smith, C and Trzaska, J (2015) Counseling through images: using photography to guide the counseling process and achieve treatment goods. *Journal of Creativity in Mental Health, 7* (4): 310–29.

Glass, N, Moss, C and Ogile, R (2012) A person-centred lifestyle change intervention model: working with older people experiencing chronic illness. *International Journal of Nursing Practice, 18* (4): 379–87.

Goffman, E (2009) *Stigma: Notes on the Management of Spoiled Identity.* New York: Simon and Schuster.

Goldman, S, Brettle, A and McAndrew, S (2016) A client focused perspective of the effectiveness of Counselling for Depression (CfD). *Counselling and Psychotherapy Research, 16* (4): 288–97.

Gomez-Urquiza, J, Hueso-Montoro, G, Urquiza-Olmo, J et al. (2016) A randomized controlled trial of the effect of a photographic display with and without music on pre-operative anxiety. *Journal of Advanced Nursing, 72* (7): 1666–76.

Gorsky, M (2013) 'Searching for the people in charge': appraising the 1983 Griffiths NHS Management Inquiry. *Medical History, 57* (1): 87–107.

Grohmann, B, Espin, S and Gucciardi, E (2017) Patients' experiences of diabetes education teams integration into primary care. *Canadian Family Physician, 63* (2): e128–e136.

Gunn, D and Mansell, P (2012) Glycaemic control and weight 7 years after Dose Adjustment for Normal Eating (DAFNE) structured education in type 1 diabetes. *Diabetic Medicine, 29* (6): 807–12.

Hakanson, C and Ohlen, J (2015) Meanings and experiential outcomes of bodily care in a specialist palliative context. *Palliative and Supportive Care, 13* (3): 625–33.

Hakanson, C, Sandberg, J, Ekstedt, M et al. (2016) Providing palliative care in a Swedish support home for people who are homeless. *Qualitative Health Research, 26* (9): 1252–62.

Harrison, S and McDonald, R (2007) *The Politics of Healthcare in Britain.* London: SAGE.

Hassan, H, Pinches, A, Picton, S et al. (2017) Survival rates and prognostic predictors of high grade brain stem gliomas in childhood: a systematic review and meta-analysis. *Journal of Neuro-Oncology, 135* (1): 13–20.

Health Education England (Willis) (2018) *Raising the Bar: Shape of Caring.* Available online at: www.hee.nhs/sites/default/files/…/2348-Shape-of-caring-review-FINAL.pdf

Heran, B, Chen, J, Ebrahim, S et al. (2011) Exercise-based cardiac rehabilitation for coronary heart disease. *The Cochrane Database of Systematic Reviews,* July 6; 7: CD001800.

Hermans, H, Beekman, A, Aartjan, T and Evenhuis, H (2014) Comparison of anxiety as reported by older people with intellectual disabilities and by older people with normal intelligence. *American Journal of Geriatric Psychiatry, 22* (12): 1391–8.

Hermans, H, Wieland, J, Jelluma, N et al. (2013) Reliability and validity of the Dutch version of the Glasgow Anxiety Scale for people with an intellectual disability (GAS-ID). *Journal of Intellectual Disability Research, 57* (8): 728–36.

Herzberg, F (1966) *Work and the Nature of Man.* New York: World Publishing.

Hoffmaster, B (2011) The rationality and morality of dying children. *The Hastings Centre Report, 41* (6): 30–42.

Hollins, S, Avis, A, Cheverton, S et al. (2015) *Going to Hospital.* London: Books Beyond Words.

Hopton, A, Eldred, J and MacPherson, H (2014) Patients' experiences of acupuncture and counselling for depression and comorbid pain: a qualitative study nested within a randomized controlled trial. *BMJ Open, 4*: e005144: doi: 10.1136/bmjopen-2014-00514-4

Horigan, G, Davies, M, Findlay-White, F, et al. (2017) Systematic review or meta-analysis: reasons why patients referred to diabetes education programmes choose not to attend. A systematic review. *Diabetic Medicine, 34* (1): 14–26.

Howell, D, Hart, R, Smith, A et al. (2018) Myeloma: patient accounts of their pathways to diagnosis. *PLOS One, 13* (4): doi: 10.1371/journal.pone.0194788

Ikard, R, Snyder, R and Roumic, C (2013) Postoperative morbidity and mortality among Veterans Health Administration patients undergoing surgical resection for large bowel polyps. *Digestive Surgery, 30* (4–6): 394–400.

Isaksson, A and Ahlström, G (2008) Managing chronic sorrow: experiences of patients with multiple sclerosis. *The Journal of Neuroscience Nursing, 40* (3): 180–92.

Jurecic, A (2012) *Illness as a Narrative.* Pittsburg: University of Pittsburg Press.

Keefer, A, Kreiser, N, Singh, V et al. (2016) Intolerance of uncertainty predicts anxiety outcomes following CBT in youth with Autistic Spectrum Disorder. *Journal of Autism and Development Disorders, 47* (12): 3949–58.

Kelly, M, Morse, J, Stover, A et al. (2011) Describing depression: congruence between patient experiences and clinical assessments. *British Journal of Clinical Psychology, 50* (1): 46–66.

Khan, N (2018) Coronary artery stents Part 1. *British Journal of Cardiac Nursing, 13* (4): doi: 10.12968/bjca.2018.13.4.168

Kim, H (2015) *The Essence of Nursing Practice.* New York: Springer Publishing Company.

Klinke, M, Wilson, M, Hafssteinnsdottir, T et al. (2013) Recognizing new perspectives in eating difficulties following a stroke: a concept analysis. *Disability and Rehabilitation, 35* (17): 1491–500.

Kornelsen, J, Atkins, C, Brownell, K et al. (2015) The meaning of patient experiences of medically unexplained physical symptoms. *Qualitative Health Research, 26* (3): 367–76.

Kragh, M, Moller, D, Wihlborg, C et al. (2017) Experiences of wake and light therapy in patients with depression: a qualitative study. *International Journal of Mental Health Nursing, 26* (2): 170–80.

Kulick, D (2018) *Heart Attack Treatment.* Medicinenet.com. Available online at: www.medicinenet.com/heart_attack_treatment/article.htm

Kwok, C, Bates, K and Ng, E (2016) Managing and sustaining an ageing nursing workforce: identifying opportunities and best practices within collective agreements. *Journal of Nursing Management, 24* (4): 500–11.

Laursen, D, Frølich, A and Christensen, U (2017a) Patients' perception of disease and experience with type 2 diabetes patient education in Denmark. *Scandinavian Journal of Caring Sciences, 31* (4): 1039–47.

Laursen, D, Christensen, K, Christensen, U and Frølich, A (2017b) Assessment of short and long term outcomes of diabetes patient education using the health education impact questionnaire (HeiQ). *BMC Research Notes, 10* (1): 213, doi: 10.1186/s13104-017-2536-6

Leaver, A, Wade, B, Vasavada, M et al. (2018) Fronto-temporal connectivity predicts ECT outcome in major depression. *Frontiers of Psychiatry, 9*: doi: 10.3389/fpsyt.2018.00092

Leplege, A, Gzil, F, Cammelli, M et al. (2007) Person-centredness: conceptual and historical perspectives. *Disability and Rehabilitation, 29* (20–21): 1555–65.

Lim, S, Chan, S, Lai, J et al. (2015) A randomized controlled trial examining the effectiveness of a stoma psychosocial intervention programme on the outcomes of colorectal patients with a stoma. *Journal of Advanced Nursing, 71* (6): 1310–23.

Lorentzen, S and Ruud, T (2014) Group therapy in public mental health services: approaches, patients and group therapists. *Journal of Psychiatric and Mental Health Nursing, 21* (3): 219–25.

Ludman, E, Peterson, D, Katon, W et al. (2013) Improving confidence for self care in patients with depression and chronic illness. *Behavioural Medicine, 39* (1): 1–6.

McCormack, B and McCance, T (2017) *Person-Centred Practice in Nursing and Health Care: Theory and Practice* (2nd edition). Chichester: Wiley/Blackwell.

McDowell, J and MacRury, S (2015) Structured diabetes patient education in Scotland. *Practical Diabetes, 32* (1): 24–8, doi: 10.1002/pdi.1916

McGreevy, J (2015) Dementia and the person-centred care approach. *Nursing Older People, 27* (8): 27–31.

McKenzie, S, Nelson, R, Mailey, B et al. (2011) Adjuvant chemotherapy improves survival in patients with American Joint Committee on Cancer Stage II colon cancer. *Cancer, 117* (24): 5493–9.

McMahon, S, Ades, P and Thompson, P (2017) The role of cardiac rehabilitation in patients with heart disease. *Trends in Cardiovascular Medicine, 27* (6): 420–5.

Mind (2018) *How Common Are Mental Health Problems?* Available online at: www.mind.org.uk/…/statistics…/how-common-are-mental-health-problems

Mitchell, G, Senior, H, Rhee, J et al. (2017) Using intuition or a formal palliative care needs assessment screening process in general practice to predict death within 12 months: a randomized controlled trial. *Palliative Medicine, 32* (2): 384–94.

Moghei, M, Turk-Adawi, K, Isarinuwatchai, W et al. (2017) Cardiac rehabilitation costs. *International Journal of Cardiology, 244*: 322–8.

Mold, A (2015) *Making the Patient-Consumer: Patient Organisations and Health Consumerism in Britain*. Manchester: Manchester University Press.

Morgan, A (2016) Identity and the health information consumer: a research agenda. *Health and Medicine, 5* (1): 1–5.

MS Society (2018) *What Is MS?* Available online at: www.mssociety.org.uk

Murray, J (2017) *Multiple Sclerosis: A Guide for the Newly Diagnosed* (5th edition). New York: Demos Medical Publishing.

National Institute for Health and Care Excellence (NICE) (2009) *Depression in Adults: Recognition and Management. Clinical Guideline (CG 90) updated April 2018*. Available online at: www.nice.org.uk/search?q=cg90

National Institute for Health and Care Excellence (NICE) (2016) *Multiple Sclerosis Quality Standard QS108*. Available online at: www.NICE.org.uk

Nelson, J and Harwood, H (2011) Learning disabilities and anxiety: a meta-analysis. *Journal of Learning Disabilities, 44* (1): 3–17.

Newman, J and Vidler, E (2006) Discriminating customers, responsible patients, empowered users. *Journal of Social Policy, 35* (2): 193–209.

NHS England (2014) *Five Year Forward View (5YFV)*. Available online at: www.england.nhs.uk/wp-content/uploads/2014/10/5yfv-web.pdf

NHS England (2017) *Next Steps on the NHS Five Year Forward View*. Available online at: www.england.nhs.uk/publications/next-steps-on-the-five-year-forward-view

NHS England (2018) *Patient Activation: People's Ability to Manage Their Own Health and Wellbeing*. Available online at: www.england.nhs.uk/ourwork/patientparticipation/self.../patient-activation

Nickerson, M and Marrie, R (2013) The multiple sclerosis relapse experience: patient reported outcomes from the North American Research Committee Scheme (NARCOMS) registry. *BMC Neurology, 13*: 119, doi: 10.1186/1471-2377-13-119

Northway, R, Rees, S, Davies, M et al. (2017) Hospital passports, patient safety and person-centred care: a review of documents currently used for people with intellectual disabilities in the UK. *Journal of Clinical Nursing, 26* (23–24): 23–4.

Nursing and Midwifery Council (NMC) (2015) *The Code: Professional Standards of Practice and Behavior for Nurses and Midwives*. Available online at: www.nmc.org.uk/globalassets/sitedocument/nmc-publications/nmc-code.pdf

Nystrom, M and Nystrom, M (2007) Patient's experiences of recurrent depression. *Issues of Mental Health Nursing, 28* (7): 673–90.

Oermann, M, McHugh, N, Dietrich, J et al. (1983) After a tracheostomy: patients describe their sensations. *Cancer Nursing, 6* (5): 361–6.

Oeseburg, B and Abma, T (2006) Care as a mutual endeavor: experiences of a multiple sclerosis patient and her healthcare professionals. *Medicine, Health Care and Philosophy, 9* (3): 349–57.

O'Hara, B, McGill, B and Phongsaven, P (2015) Preventative health coaching: is there room to be more prescriptive? *International Journal of Health Promotion and Education, 54* (2): 82–94.

Ohlen, J, Reimer-Kirkham, S, Astle, B et al. (2017) Person-centred care didactics: inquired in the context of palliative care. *Nursing Philosophy, 18* (4): e12177, doi.rcn.idm.oclc.org/10.1111/nup.12177

Olaug, L and Robson, C (2017) 'It's incredible how much I've had to fight: negotiating medical uncertainty in clinical encounters. *International Journal of Qualitative Studies on Health and Well-being, 12* (1): 1–13.

Oliver, D (2017) Choosing to be honest about patient choice. *BMJ (British Medical Journal), 357*: j1829, doi: 10.1136/bmj.j1829

Olkiewicz, M and Bober, B (2015) Role of quality in healthcare service provision process. *Progress in Health Sciences, 5* (2): 41–53.

Olsen, J (2014) Health coaching: a concept analysis. *Nursing Forum, 49* (1): 18–29.

Olsson, L and Ung, E (2012) Efficacy of person-centred care as an intervention in a controlled trial: a systematic review. *Journal of Clinical Nursing, 22* (3–4): 456–65.

Owen, R (2014) *Living with the Enemy: Coping with the Stress of Chronic Illness using CBT, Mindfulness and Acceptance.* Abingdon: Routledge.

Parsons, T (1951) *The Social System.* London: Tavistock Publications.

Pearce, Z (2014) *Type 1 Diabetes: Causes, Treatment and Potential Complications.* New York: Nova Science Publishers.

Perti, M, Heney, D, Collier, S et al. (2014) Predictors of fatigue in cancer patients before and after chemotherapy. *Journal of Health Psychology, 19* (6): 699–710.

Polit, B and Feiring, M (2016) Challenges in the nurses role in rehabilitation contexts. *Journal of Clinical Nursing, 26* (19–20), doi: 10.1111/jocn.13674

Pols, A, Schipper, K, Overkamp, D et al. (2017) Process evaluation of a stepped-care program to prevent depression in primary care: patients' and practice nurses' experiences. *BMC Family Practice, 18* (1): 26, doi: 10.1186/s12875-017-0583-7

Price, B (2015) Helping patients to learn about self-management. *Nursing Standard, 30* (2): 51–60.

Price, B (2017a) Developing patient rapport, trust and therapeutic relationships. *Nursing Standard, 31* (50): 52–63.

Price, B (2017b) How to write up a reflective practice case study. *Primary Health Care, 27* (9): 35–42, doi: 10.7748/phc.2017.e1328

Price, B (2017c) Managing patients' anxiety about planned medical interventions. *Nursing Standard, 31* (47): 53–63.

Ramanathan, M, Mackay, G, Platt, J et al. (2015) The impact of open versus laproscopic resection for colon cancer on C-reactive protein concentrations as a predictor of postoperative infective complications. *Annals of Surgical Oncology, 22* (3): 938–43.

Rankin, J (2015) The rhetoric of patient and family-centred care: an institutional ethnography into what actually happens. *Journal of Advanced Nursing, 71* (3): 526–34.

Reed, F, Fitzgerald, L and Bish, M (2017) Rural district nursing experiences of successful advocacy for person-centred end-of-life choice. *Journal of Holistic Nursing, 35* (2): 151–64.

Reid, K, Smiley, E and Cooper, E (2011) Prevalence and associations of anxiety disorders in adults with intellectual disabilities. *Journal of Intellectual Disability Research, 55* (2): 172–81.

Richards, B (2017) Caring for children with autism spectrum condition in paediatric emergency departments. *Emergency Nurse, 25* (4): 30–4.

Riding, S, Glendening, N and Heaslip, V (2017) Real world challenges in delivering person-centred care: a community-based case study. *British Journal of Community Nursing, 22* (8): 391–6.

Rivett, G (1998) *From Cradle to Grave: the History of the NHS 1948–1987 and 1988 Onwards.* Blurb Books (ebook). Available online at: www.Blurb.co.uk

Roberts, D (2013) *Psychosocial Nursing Care: A Guide to Nursing the Whole Person.* Maidenhead: Open University Press.

Rogers, E, Cannon, A, Zabrowski, K and Paul, S (2016) Early recognition and management of brain tumours in children. *Nursing Standard, 31* (1): 42–9.

Rosa, W (2014) Intertwined narratives of the human caring story. *Creative Nursing, 20* (3): 171–3.

Rose, P and Yates, P (2015) Patients' outcomes related to person-centred nursing care in radiation oncology: a case study. *European Journal of Oncology Nursing, 19* (6): 731–9.

Royal College of Psychiatrists (2009) *Antidepressants: Key Facts from the Royal College of Psychiatrists.* Available online at: www.rcpsych.ac.uk/pdf/antidepressants.pdf

Salmon, N (2017) British people rank among the most depressed people in Western World. *The Independent,* 13 September. Available online at: www.independent.co.uk/news/uk/home-news/british-people-depression-west-mental-health-uk-oecd-europe-scandinavia-women-more-men-a7945321.html

Sanders, P and Hill, A (2014) *Counselling for Depression: A Person-Centred and Experiential Approach to Practice.* London: SAGE.

Sanderson, H (2014) *Person-Centred Teams: A Practical Guide to Delivering Personalization Through Effective Teamwork.* London: Jessica Kingsley Publishing.

Satekova, L, Ziakova, K and Zelenikova, R (2017) Predictive validity of the Braden scale, Norton scale and Waterlow scale in the Czech Republic. *International Journal of Nursing Practice, 23*(1): e12499, doi: 10.1111/ijn.12499

Schaepe, C and Ewers, M (2017) 'I need complete trust in nurses': home mechanical ventilated patients' perceptions of safety. *Scandinavian Journal of Caring Sciences, 31* (4): 948–56.

Schopf, A, Ullrich, A, Nagi, M et al. (2015) Group health education in inpatient rehabilitation: patients' role perceptions. *Health Education Journal, 75* (3): 289–305.

Schopfer, D and Forman, D (2016) Cardiac rehabilitation in older adults. *Canadian Journal of Cardiology, 32* (9): 1088–96.

Segal, J (2017) *The Trouble with Illness: How Illness and Disability Affect Relationships.* London: Jessica Kingsley Publishing.

Sharma, T, Bamford, M and Dodman, D (2015) Person-centred care: an overview of reviews. *Contemporary Nurse, 51* (2–3): 107–20.

Sharp, S, McAllister, M and Broadbent, M (2016) The vital blend of clinical competence and compassion: how patients experience person-centred care. *Contemporary Nurse, 52* (2–3): 300–12.

Shea, M (2015) Determined persistence: achieving and sustaining job satisfaction among nurse practitioners. *Journal of American Association of Nurse Practitioners, 27* (1): 31–8.

Sheridan, N, Kenealy, T, Schmidt-Busby, J et al. (2012) Patients' engagement in primacy care: powerlessness and compounding jeopardy – a qualitative study. *Health Expectations, 18* (1): 32–43.

Shrank, W (2017) Primary care practice transformation and the rise of consumerism. *Journal of General Internal Medicine, 32* (4): 387–91.

Sillence, E, Hardy, C, Briggs, P et al. (2016) How do carers of people with multiple sclerosis engage with websites containing the personal experiences of other carers and patients. *Health Informatics Journal, 22* (4): 1045–54.

Skundberg-Kletthagen, H, Wangenstein, S, Hall-Lord, M et al. (2014) Relatives of patients with depression: experiences of everyday life. *Scandinavian Journal of Caring Sciences, 28* (3): 564–71.

Slomic, M, Christiansen, B, Soberg, H et al. (2016) User involvement and experiential knowledge in interprofessional rehabilitation: a grounded theory study. *BMC Health Services Research, 16* (1): 547, doi: 10.1186/s12913-016-1808-5

Snow, R, Humphrey, C and Sandall, J (2013) What happens when patients know more than their doctors? Experiences of health interactions after diabetes patient education. A qualitative patient analysis. *BMJ Open, 3*: e003583, doi: 10.1136/bmjopen-2013-003585

Snow, R, Sandall, J and Humphrey, C (2014) Use of clinical targets in diabetes patient education: qualitative analysis of the expectations and impact of a structured self-management programme in type 1 diabetes. *Diabetic Medicine, 31* (6): 733–8.

Solheim, A, Mygland, A and Ljostad, U (2017) Quality of multiple sclerosis outpatient health care services with focus on patient reported experiences. *BMC Research Notes, 10*: 250, doi: 10.1186/s13104-017-2568-y

Sox, H and Stewart, W (2015) Algorithms, clinical practice guidelines and standardized clinical assessment and management plans: evidence-based patient management standards in evolution. *Academic Medicine, 90* (20): 129–32.

Spouse, J (2000) An impossible dream? Images of nursing held by pre-registration students and their effect on sustaining motivation to become nurses. *Journal of Advanced Nursing, 32* (3): 730–9.

Stanek, S (2017) Goals of care: a concept clarification. *Journal of Advanced Nursing, 73* (6): 1302–14.

Stirk, S and Sanderson, H (2012) *Creating Person-Centred Organisations: Managing Change in Health and Social Care.* London: Jessica Kingsley Publishers.

Stone, L (2014) Blame, shame and hopelessness: medically unexplained symptoms and the 'heartsink' experience. *Australian Family Physician, 43* (4): 191–5.

Strohbuecker, B, Eisemann, Y, Galusko, M et al. (2011) Palliative care needs of chronically ill nursing home residents in Germany: focusing on living, not dying. *International Journal of Palliative Nursing, 17* (1): 27–34.

Sustersic, M, Gauchet, A, Foote, A et al. (2017) How best to use and evaluate patient information leaflets given during a consultation: a systematic review of literature reviews. *Health Expectations, 20* (4): 531–42, doi: 10.1111/hex.12487

Taipale, J (2014) *Phenomenology and Embodiment: Husserl and the Constitution of Subjectivity.* Evanston, IL: Northwestern University Press.

Talking Sense (2018) *Counselling for Depression: Rotherham, Doncaster and South Humber NHS Foundation Trust. Improving Access to Psychological Therapies (IAPT).* Available online at: www.talkingsense.org/how-we-can…therapy/…therapy/counselling-for-depression

Thomas, R, Phillips, M and Hamilton, R (2018) Pain management in the pediatric palliative care population. *Journal of Nursing Scholarship, 50* (4): 375–82.

Tiller, S, Leger-Caldwell, L, O'Farrell, P et al. (2013) Cardiac rehabilitation beginning at the bedside. *Journal of Cardiopulmonary Rehabilitation and Prevention, 33* (3): 180–4.

Tonnessen, S, Ursin, G and Brinchmann, B (2017) Care-manager's professional choices: ethical dilemmas and conflicting expectations. *BMC Health Service Research, 17:* 630, doi. org/10.1186/s12913-017-2578-4

Traynor, M (1999) *Managerialism and Nursing: Beyond Oppression and Profession.* Abingdon: Routledge.

Van der Aa, H, Van Rens, G, Comijs, H et al. (2015) Stepped care for depression and anxiety in visually impaired older adults: multicenter randomized controlled trial. *BMJ, 351:* h6127, doi: 10.1136/bmj.h6127

Van Veer-Tazelaar, P, Van Marwijk, H, Van Oppen, P et al. (2009) Stepped-care prevention of anxiety and depression in late life: a randomized controlled trial. *Archives of General Psychiatry, 66* (3): 297–304.

Vidovic, V, Rovazdi, M, Silvar, S et al. (2014) Pain syndromes in multiple sclerosis patients – patient experience at Lipik Special Hospital for Medical Rehabilitation. *Acta Clinica Croatia, 53* (4): 405–10.

Waterworth, S, Arroll, B, Raphael, D et al. (2015) A qualitative study of nurses' clinical experience in recognizing low mood and depression in older patients with multiple long term conditions. *Journal of Clinical Nursing, 24* (17–18): 2562–70.

Way, S and Scammell, J (2016) Humanising midwifery care. *The Practising Midwife, 19* (3): 27–9.

Wazni, L and Gifford, W (2017) Addressing physical health needs of individuals with schizophrenia using Orem's model. *Journal of Holistic Nursing, 35* (3): doi: 10.1177/0898010116658366

Weeks, J, Catalano, P, Cronin, A et al. (2012) Patients' expectations about effects of chemotherapy for advanced cancer. *The New England Journal of Medicine, 367* (17): 1616–25.

Weiner, B (2010) The development of an attribution-based theory of motivation: a history of ideas. *Educational Psychologist, 45* (1): 28–36.

Welch, E (2018) *The NHS at 70: A Living History.* Barnsley: Pen and Sword History.

West, R, Jones, D and Henderson, A (2012) Rehabilitation after myocardial infarction trial (RAMIT): multi centre randomized controlled trial of comprehensive cardiac rehabilitation in patients following acute myocardial infarction. *Heart, 98* (8): 637–44.

Whittaker, S, Baldwin, T, Tahir, M et al. (2012) Public knowledge of the symptoms of myocardial infarction: a street survey in Birmingham England. *Family Practice, 29* (2): 168–73.

Wigert, H and Wikström, A (2014) Organising personalized care in paediatric diabetes: multidisciplinary teams, long-term relationships and adequate documentation. *BMC Research Notes, 7:* 72, doi: 10.1186/1756-0500-7-72

Williams, L, O'Connor, R, Grubb, N and O'Carroll, R (2011) Type D personality predicts poor medication adherence in myocardial infarction patients. *Psychology and Health, 26* (6): 703–12.

Wlodarcyzk, D (2017) Optimism and hope as predictors of subjective health in post myocardial infarction patients: a comparison of the role of coping strategies.*Journal of Health Psychology, 22* (3): 336–46.

Wood, I and Garner, M (2012) *Initial Management of Acute Medical Patients: A Guide for Nurses and Healthcare Practitioners* (2nd edition). Chichester: Wiley Blackwell.

Index